A Medical Expert's Guide to Self-Transform~~~~~~~ ~~~~evity

Th

HAPPINESS
REVOLUTION

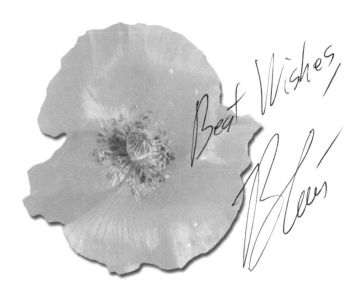

Best Wishes,

CREATING BALANCE
AND HARMONY
IN YOUR LIFE

BLAIR LEWIS, P.A.

The Happiness Revolution
Creating Balance and Harmony in Your Life

A Medical Expert's Guide to Self-Transformation
and Longevity

Published by:
Alive and Healthy Institute Press
www.AliveandHealthy.com

Disclaimer:
While the following text may change your paradigm about how disease can be treated, cured and managed, it is not intended to substitute for professional medical care. This book is not intended to treat, diagnose, or prescribe. Instead, this text represents a body of knowledge thousands of years old that has been applied to modern times. The information contained herein may be used according to your good common sense or as advised by a health care professional.

ISBN 13: 978-0-9789566-0-8
ISBN 10: 0-9789566-0-5
Printed in Korea

Library of Congress Cataloging in Publication Data

Lewis, Blair.
        The Happiness Revolution
        P.cm.
        Includes Index
        ISBN 978-0-9789566-0-8
        1. Self-Help. 2. Holistic Health 3. Yoga
        4. Psychology 5. Ayurveda

Cover Design by www.Bookcovers.com
Photographs by Deven Karvelas, www.DevPhotos.com
Illustrations by Jeff Hiser, www.HiserIllustrated.com

Table of Contents

Dedication

It was my mom who taught me to write. I was then inspired to become a writer by Mrs. Small's reading of A Wrinkle in Time to my fifth-grade class. Mom saw this coming. A year earlier she encouraged me to start a diary about my life, the writings of which continue today, some 40 years later.

Before motherhood, she was an English teacher. My pre-teen writing ineptitude would pull her out of early retirement and I became her most desperate pupil. She and I spent many hours writing together on the old dining room table kept in the basement family room. It was in that room where Mom and Dad read us Robert Louis Stevenson's Treasure Island and Johanna Spyri's Heidi. It was a Sunday night ritual every winter throughout elementary school: A blazing fire in the fireplace, a hot thick stew or grilled steak for dinner and us kids listening to great tales as we snuggled in front of the fireplace.

On Sunday nights I would stow away on a Mississippi raft with Huck and Tom; live in a tree house with the Swiss Family Robinson; and puzzle over solitude with Robinson Crusoe. My parents knew how to use words to build picturesque worlds in our minds. When my mind was blank from the struggles of high school term-paper-phobia, my mother would remind me of the fireside stories of my childhood. Immediately I could feel the warmth of the crackling wood and the words would start to flow again onto the paper.

Knowing that I am dedicating this book to my mother, I am misty with memories of how we wrote some of the greatest vaudeville jokes and sketches on that old table. Our whole family loved and continues to love the theater. Musicals and comedies are the top of the heap. As I share with you the stories of my family and patients, I hope you find the joy and comfort that my boyhood found in great books snuggling by the fire.

This book is written in loving gratitude to Barbara Ann Lewis, my mother, and her only brother, Philip Halfaker, who constantly inspired adventure in my soul. Thank you, Mom. May my writings honor your teachings.

Your loving son,

Blair

❀   ❀   ❀

My mom would like you to know what to read to your kids. First, start reading to them before they are born and make sure that by the time they finish the fifth grade they have read:

Louisa May Alcott's *Little Women*
J.M. Barrie's *Peter Pan*
William Howard Armstrong's *Sounder*
L. Frank Baum's *The Wizard of Oz*
Frances Hodgson Burnett's *The Secret Garden*
Roald Dahl's *Charlie and the Chocolate Factory*
Rudyard Kipling's *The Jungle Book*
C. S. Lewis' *The Lion, the Witch, and the Wardrobe*
Astrid Lindgren's *Pippi Longstocking*
A.A. Milne's *The House at Pooh Corner*
L.M. Montgomery's *Anne of Green Gables*
Anna Sewell's *Black Beauty*
Robert Louis Stevenson's *Treasure Island*
Johanna Spyri's *Heidi*
J.R.R. Tolkien's *The Hobbit*
E.B. White's *Charlotte's Web*
Mark Twain's *The Adventures of Tom Sawyer* and *Huckleberry Finn*

She thought this list would get you started. Ask your librarian for more titles and suggestions. Mom would be so happy if you did.

Introduction

E ver notice how we are told over and over that we will become happy by buying the products advertisers are selling? If it is not a product, then it is an experience, a destination, or sometimes even a medication. Regardless, modern society leads us to believe that the source of happiness is external and expensive.

You know that this is not true. Yet, we are all human. We would all like a "quick fix," even if, at some level, we're aware that we're indulging in wishful thinking. So, as we live our hurried, stressful, overscheduled lives, we continue to purchase the illusion of joy – and thus, we are disappointed again and again.

This book is filled with immediate actions that will help you connect to the true source of happiness that lies within you. There is a science to happiness as there is to health and longevity. It is a science that includes biochemistry and physiology, but more importantly it addresses the lifestyle, determination and self-esteem of the seeker. It does not require you to purchase anything, but it does require you to set aside a few minutes each day just for you. You will recognize your own worth and the value of being happy – happy in a manner that embraces disappointment as well as success.

My hunch is that you are reading these pages because you are looking to improve your life or the life of someone you love. I am not going to disappoint you. Instead of pop psychology and New Age psycho-babble, let's go with what works – with techniques that anybody can understand. (I can feel your relief!)

Modern medicine does not recognize happiness as its goal. That's too bad. In my experience, happiness is *the* key to good health. When patients walk into my office, I can easily correlate their health with their levels of happiness. It is an obvious connection. When I see patients who do not have high levels of happiness, there are equivalent deficits somewhere in their general health status. To help them, I always begin with simple strategies that will bring quick success.

> *Happiness is the key to good health.*

When you start your journey to happiness by making the best use of things that you know and understand, success comes easily and quickly. I see this truth played out over and over with my patients. Once they understand that there is a biological and lifestyle foundation for true happiness, I then teach them how to sleep, eat, breathe and think properly. Believe it or not, these simple things are the most important pillars of a happy person. When you learn to sleep in a manner that provides deep rest and you wake up delighted and ready to go, it will be obvious that happiness is within your grasp. When you know which foods are great for your body and mind, then you will be able to take incredibly good care of yourself and your loved ones. When the relationship between inspiration (inhaling) and feeling inspired is experienced, then the significance of how you breathe will instantly be a high priority. And lastly, *thinking* is key. Developing a personal philosophy that allows you to face every life event with courage and compassion is essential to living the life of a happy and helpful person.

Sleeping, breathing, eating, thinking – these are the kinds of practical things that, when done well, will amplify happiness in your life and prevent you from succumbing to the lure of enticing commercials and excess consumerism. This book proposes a happiness that is everlasting and incorruptible.

When I encountered challenging times, Pandit Rajmani Tigunait, PhD., my teacher of Ayurveda and meditation, often told me that the only things standing between me and everlasting happiness were the noise and the aberrations in my body, breath, and mind. He said, "If you design your life around the goal of happiness, then your capacity to help and serve others will eventually become unlimited, for only with limitless joy and enthusiasm can you have the courage to do what needs to be done and the mental clarity to see what needs to be done."

To shift life events in your favor, you will need to have your entire operating system supporting *you*, not your willpower alone. Your determination must also be supported by a sound philosophy, a healthy diet, and a simple exercise program. The internal programming of your mind must be based on a well-selected personal philosophy that reflects your goals and purpose. Your diet must not be littered with foods and beverages known to cause dullness or agitation. You can choose foods and seasonings that will sustain you in a manner that enhances your mental clarity, compassion, and intuition. Furthermore, your exercise program and breathing habits can become useful aids in your journey to finding invincible happiness. This book will help you discover these techniques and create a reliable mind and body so that happiness may blossom and flourish.

This book will help you self-select therapies that you can immediately apply to your life. You will begin by defining your constitution – your base of needs and wants that dominate your physiology and desires. Ayurvedic medicine provides that finest means for this analysis. Then you will explore 10 main principles for selecting optimal behaviors within the privacy of your own mind and in society. Next comes food and fitness, followed by the most common homeopathic remedies for stress management. The science of sleep, rest and relaxation will be explored in detail. These techniques will bolster your mental clarity and eliminate fatigue. Yoga offers an amazing method for creating more space in your day – what would your life be like if you could create more time for yourself, your job and your family? Chapter Nine will show you how.

Next comes time management – an absolutely essential skill in the pursuit of happiness. Then you will learn how to use contemplation and meditation as a means to refine your ability to listen to your conscience. And the book concludes with a discussion on mentorship, your ancestors and finally, love and longevity. The sages state that love supercedes all the laws of karma and thus becomes the finest force for self-transformation and healing. You will learn how to do it all.

If you want to create courage, enthusiasm and limitless joy in your life, then you have come to the right book. Welcome. I wish you a rich, fruitful journey and am honored to be a part of it all.

A Personal Note

In the following pages you are going to meet many people and patients that helped shape my career and my personal life. Three of them merit a special introduction.

First is Swami Rama, my spiritual teacher, who inspired me to believe that healing and transformation are possible for all people, including myself. He is the founder of the Himalayan Institute, which is based in Honesdale, Pennsylvania, and has branches throughout the world. I commonly refer to him as Swamiji.

Second is Pandit Rajmani Tigunait, PhD., the successor to Swami Rama and the current Spiritual Head of the Himalayan Institute. For over 25 years he has been my teacher, role model and best friend. Pandit Rajmani, whom I call 'Panditji,' continues to inspire and instruct me in the science of yoga, tantra and Ayurveda. Without his living presence, this book would not exist.

And finally, Karen Lewis, was my wife for almost two decades and continues to nurture and befriend me. Together and individually, we do our best to help each other and all whom we meet.

A Prelude

A great yogi, named Dattatreya, in answering his student, Parashurama, gave the following insight on the fast-track to happiness: To achieve happiness, you must find people who have attained a level of joy that supersedes all others. He says that it begins with the company of mentors and coaches who have achieved the goal that you are now pursuing.

People may expect their good deeds to help diminish their conflicts and problems, but sometimes this result does not seem to manifest itself. During that time, the seeker of happiness may start to wonder why those who perform good actions appear to suffer throughout life, while selfish people appear to be happy and successful. These momentary glimpses can mislead you if you are unable to gain the counsel of wise mentors. That is why coming into the company of the wise is a critical juncture in the evolution of your journey. Through this relationship, your knowledge begins to mature as your mentors broaden your self-understanding.

Behind every action is the desire to attain happiness – the clarity of this fact may or may not be readily apparent. But the true nature of happiness is self-evident, and thus, your mentors must teach you the inward method of this discovery. The knowledge you are seeking can only be revealed with an inward, one-pointed mind. There is no other way, because it has to come from within you. That is why many ancient texts cheer your efforts, saying "Look within; Seek within; Find within!" No one outside of you can prove your existence to you. Only through non-attachment can you enjoy the freedom to dive deep into your self and attain complete liberation from the tyranny of your mind and senses. When you realize that your essential nature is indestructible, your habit of uselessly defending yourself will diminish. When you are misunderstood by others, you will no longer become defensive and disappointed. When your mind is free from all conflicting thoughts, then you achieve the one-pointedness necessary to traverse the depths of your mind and soul. This is the journey back to your essential nature of peace, happiness and wisdom.

The mind is the cause of both bondage and liberation. That is why you must protect your mind at all costs from confusion and despair. Befriend and guide your mind back to its source. That is where you will find the happiness you seek.

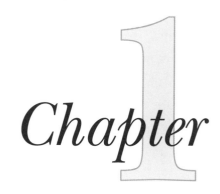

Chapter

Sturdy Body and Stable Mind

Your mind and body are your greatest friends and allies. If this is true, then why does your mind torment you and your body have so many requests? It would seem that these "friends" are more a distraction in life and are very high maintenance. It is the premise of this book that happiness and health are not only linked, they are inherently intertwined. When this is not your experience, happiness has not forsaken you, rather you have forsaken it. Your abandonment of joy is unintentional, and commonly, accidental. When you regain the stability of your mind and the sturdiness of your body, health and happiness return in full force. This is what I have learned, but this is not how my life began.

I began, like all of us, curious, slightly clueless, and easily distracted by this amazing world. My mind was full of impulses flowing from an unknown source that I never thought to question or validate. In my adult years, I trained in medicine as a physician assistant. Learning the physiology of the body was fascinating but not helpful in my pursuit of happiness. My definition of my goal – happiness – was based on an ever-expanding continuum of experience and thought.

I was really lost in my pursuit. It seemed that I was a victim of too much input from my five senses – touching, smelling, seeing, tasting and hearing. If I could channel and prioritize this constant flow of stimulation and information, then maybe I could start to figure myself out.

Is it obvious to you that your senses are the most external part of your body? Your arms are only so many inches long, but your ears can grasp sounds from miles away. Your eyes can see beautiful mountain vistas looming in the distance. Fragrant aromas from the flower gardens in your neighborhood can be enjoyed from your window. When your five senses are fortified and trained, they serve as your most important allies in maintaining your inner joy.

> *Happiness has not forsaken you, rather you have forsaken it.*

I soon came to realize that you can train your senses to reveal information and solutions, or you can let them transmit fear and doubt into the deepest recesses of your mind. It is up to you to decide what your senses pay attention to and what they transport inside you. When your senses are properly trained, they can bring you everything you need to understand and enjoy this world. However, without proper barricades and fortifications, your mind will become cluttered with mundane souvenirs and useless memories instead of inspirational thoughts and useful knowledge.

OBSERVE YOUR SENSES

Your first step toward building sturdy senses begins with careful observation. The easiest way to observe your five senses is to zero-in on them in a situation that challenges and over-amplifies the sensory streaming of input into your brain. For some people, the noise and bustle of the crowds at the mall can send them running for the exit. However, on other days, those same people can enjoy the excitement of the mall. It was the sturdiness of their senses on that particular day that determined their reactions to the crowds of shoppers.

As you advance, you will also notice that your senses can vary with increasing or diminishing sensitivity and susceptibility. On days when your senses are overwhelmed, it is not because you are physically ill, but rather because your senses were not sturdy enough to handle all of the external stimulation. You can instantly see this connection in the faces of young children overwhelmed with sensory stimulation. Both you and the children can learn how to fortify your senses so that you are not upset by clamor and commotion. In this book, you will learn how to use your diet, your breath and your personal philosophy as a starting point to strengthen your senses and your reaction to the ever-changing inventory of sensory input. Gaining mastery over this aspect of your mind will provide you with the freedom to focus on the most important aspects of your day and minimize the risk of feeling overwhelmed. Sturdy senses are necessary in order to live your life fully engaged and fully present in every moment.

Bolstering your senses requires self-study. You need to understand how your mind works and how external data can ruin your day. Potentially troubling data may arise from emails, cable news shows, local gossip and common misunderstandings. When you let this external information stream in through your senses unedited and un-inspected, it muddles the purity and quiet of your mind. Like any unorganized basement or attic, your mind soon becomes filled with a hodgepodge of worldly stuff. Organized or unorganized, your mental contents constantly influence your choices, opinions and reactions. Sturdy senses act as gates and turnstiles that allow for an orderly flow of edited information to enter the privacy of your mind.

As you study your senses, you realize that there are two key players that affect the sorting of sensory data: the *buddhi* (conscience) and *ahamkara* (your ego). Your buddhi is the pure part of yourself that always gives accurate information and feedback. Your ego is the part of yourself that is always looking out for you and is concerned with self-preservation and identity. Any threat to your reputation or image is devastating to the ego. The key to having sturdy senses is to utilize your buddhi more than your ego. The buddhi only grasps what is helpful and useful and discards the useless parts. The ego, on the other hand, grasps information that is attractive and captivating, but may not be helpful in any way.

The battle between ego and buddhi is best explained in the following example. Someone might call you a bad name and your ego might retain that information in your awareness for days, weeks or even years. Such a "bad memory" may then alter your actions and contaminate your compassion. However, with a trained buddhi, when you are called that bad name, your buddhi will discard that information as unwanted and useless. You will never recall those bad words again, and thus your actions and compassion are not halted by someone's rudeness.

The more you employ the talents of your buddhi and ignore the noise of the ego, the stronger and sturdier your senses will be. When your mind no longer stores useless fancies for the ego, you will always be guided in the correct direction. This ability will become an invaluable asset in your life that cannot be revoked by anyone or anything.

SHARPENING YOUR AXE

The first step in training your mind requires you to actively participate in the process of sorting information and experiences. You need to realize exactly what sensory information your mind is receiving. When I first began to explore this sorting process, I had to actually stop what I was doing and sit down. The more willingly I allowed for this "down time," the more quickly I was able to sort this data and continue with my day. It was during this period in my life that a teacher of meditation inspired me with a story of a wood-chopping contest.

According to legend, in the great northern woods of Wisconsin there was once a contest between two wood-choppers. Whoever could chop the greatest amount of wood in eight hours would be the winner. With shiny, sharpened axes, the two contestants approached their enormous woodpiles.

From the moment the contest began, one woodsman chopped continuously. For the entire eight hours he never stopped chopping wood. The other fellow chopped for an hour and then stopped to rest for ten minutes. And then, like clockwork, he would start to chop again. At the end of the eight hours, it was the man who rested every hour who won the contest by a dramatic margin. Amazed and confused, his fellow contestant inquired about the winner's secret. Without hesitation the winner freely told him: "Every time I stopped to rest, I sharpened my axe."

You also need to stop throughout the day and take time to sharpen your mind. Your sharpened mind will not allow your ego to torment you. Once you can objectively observe your sorting process in action, you will start making better decisions quickly and feel the stress falling from your shoulders. You will develop sturdier senses. In a later chapter, I will show you which foods and beverages can further fortify your senses.

The next time someone says something unpleasant to you, actively try to find some hidden positive value in their comments instead of allowing your mind to focus only on the negative aspects. Many people have completely trained their mind to discard all positive comments and focus only on the negatives ones.

If you win a tiny goldfish at the local fair, only to have it suddenly die the following day, then it is appropriate to temporarily feel sad about your loss. However, if you are grieving for 12 years after this brief experience with the goldfish, then the mind has become too fond of disappointments, having completely forgotten your success of winning the goldfish. Everyone experiences grief, but a person on the path to happiness understands the nature of life and focuses on the positive successes and does not dwell on the momentary failures.

Once you have extracted the useful positive wisdom from every life experience, then you can discard that which is no longer useful as historical trash. Thus, you force yourself to benefit from all situations (whether they initially appear as positive or negative). Training your mind in this manner is learnable and attainable. When you live your life with a trained mind, it is impossible to become bitter or harbor ill-will toward others because you simply don't retain negative comments and useless losses of the past.

Your decision-making faculty, the buddhi, when coupled with a purified ego, creates a powerful force that can overcome the obstacles in your life. However, training your ego requires understanding the nature of life's events. The wise teachers say that every 24 hours you will go through the seasons of loss and gain, honor and insult, success and failure, reward and punishment. The magnitude of these experiences may be dramatic or minute. Regardless, this constant ebb and flow of experience reminds us that both glory and failure are fleeting. Thus, you learn to enjoy the richness of every experience. No longer will you cling to some events while hiding from others. The moment you start embracing all aspects of life is the moment when all stress evaporates. You can train your ego to incorporate this attitude into your personality. Over time, this uplifting perspective will happen as naturally as breathing. Without fear and possessiveness, stress cannot exist.

As you recognize the fluctuating nature of daily life, your sturdy, fortified senses and trained mind will filter your life experiences and recurring memories into inspiring and informative moments. When your intellect understands the basic nature of daily life – that it is always in flux – then your mind will be prepared to experience all of the seasons of life and will filter them with great ease and skill. With honesty and objectivity, you will be able to organize all sensory data in a manner that will keep you fearless and enthusiastic every moment of the day and every day of your life.

> *Without fear and possessiveness, stress cannot exist.*

CHAPTER SUMMARY

· *Happiness is your true nature. When you regain the stability of your mind and the sturdiness of your body, then health and happiness will return in full force.*

· *What you store in your mind will shape your experience of life.*

· *Your buddhi (conscience) is the guard at the gate into your mind. It can help you choose what to allow in and what to discard.*

ACTION ITEMS

· *Practice trying to distinguish between the thoughts presented by your buddhi (conscience) and the thoughts presented by your ego (see Chapter 11 for tips on how to do this).*

· *Take some breaks during your day to actively sort the input you have been receiving from your senses. Your breath will shorten as your mind and senses fill with input and matters that need attention. Take a few moments to breathe and lengthen your breath. This is a great first step into gaining the mental clarity needed to make good decisions. Your clarity will make it obvious what to store and what to discard. More information on how to sort out sensory input is discussed in a later chapter on contemplation.*

· *Practice extracting the most useful and positive wisdom from every life experience, regardless of whether the experience itself was pleasant or unpleasant.*

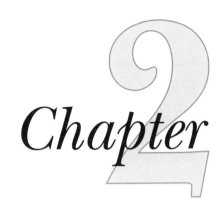

Chapter

Know Yourself
Determining Your Ayurvedic Constitution

A PRELUDE TO JOY

To find happiness *now*, you need shortcuts, direct access. To know which path to take, you must first know who you are, what you are and what resources you have available. In the next few pages I will help you understand and identify with this concept. Once you know yourself at a comprehensive level, progress can be easy and rapid. I have chosen a methodology that has stood the test of time – more than 5,000 years. This seems like a reasonable and trustworthy evaluation period. I have been studying and teaching this medical science for more than 20 years. It is called Ayurveda (pronounced I-yer-VAY-da). Don't worry if you've never heard of this ancient science. I will teach you the basic principles that will allow you to move quickly into *now*. I will provide simple surveys to help determine your body and personality type.

You must understand yourself: your body temperament, your mental and emotional reactions to stress, your preference for food seasonings (salty, sweet, sour, etc). All of these factors define your constitution. They are the most basic considerations in Ayurveda's diagnosis and treatment.

> *To know which path to take, you must first know who you are, what you are and what resources you have available.*

I have seen holistic therapies and modern medicine fail because the treatment plan was not adjusted to the constitution of the specific patient. Likewise, all of us have unknowingly violated the rules and guidelines that support our own health at a very personal level. Simple things were overlooked – encouraging thin people to fast; not encouraging larger people to exercise.

Once you know your constitutional type – more on that in a moment – then you can leap to any chapter or topic that seems most practical to you right now. I do encourage you to spend a few moments in the chapter on homeopathy – these remedies have been the miracle makers for so many of my patients and friends. If you feel incredibly stuck in your thoughts, habits and dietary choices, then homeopathic remedies may be the very shortcut that liberates you. This book will help you self-select therapies that you can immediately apply to your life. I will show you how to use food, exercise, time management, homeopathy, meditation, contemplation and relaxation to increase your confidence, productivity and joy every day.

THE BASICS

Throughout human history, the concept of self-understanding has been fundamental to virtually every culture and religion. The Greeks inscribed "Know Thyself" at the temple to Apollo in the sixth century BC. Also in that century, the Taoist sage Lao Tsu, wrote, "Those who know others are wise. Those who know themselves are enlightened."[1] According to the Gospel of Thomas, Jesus said, "When you come to know yourselves, then you will become known, and you will realize that it is you who are the sons of the living Father."[2] All of these rich traditions impart the same message: that knowing yourself is essential.

You need this self-knowledge in order to begin your journey. You must understand your physical and mental predispositions, your strengths and your weaknesses. From this foundation you can go on to understand yourself at deeper levels. The science of Ayurveda offers a methodology for beginning your self-exploration.

Ayurveda honors the diversity of all people, acknowledging that individuals have different habits, body types, food preferences, attitudes and personalities. It breaks down each individual characteristic of a person into various blends of three major categories: Vata, Pitta and Kapha. Thus, each person contains some habits and traits of each of these categories. When you know which category is most dominant in you, then you will have a better understanding of your nature.

Throughout human history, the concept of self-understanding has been fundamental to virtually every culture and religion.

When I describe the three constitutions of Vata, Pitta and Kapha, you will probably be able to immediately think of someone in your life who fits that description. Once you understand your Ayurvedic constitution, it is easy to match diet plans, sleep therapies, hatha yoga routines, and other aspects of your life to it.

The three Ayurvedic constitutions are based on the main elements of nature: space, air, earth, water, and fire. According to Ayurveda, these five elements are present in everything in varying degrees. To simplify this science, Ayurveda further generalizes the five elements into the three main constitutions. I use images to accent the main characteristics of each constitution.

THE THREE AYURVEDIC CONSTITUTIONS

The first constitution is Vata. To visualize Vata, you can imagine a thin person riding the cold, dry winds of outer space. This person is primarily composed of the elements of space and air. Thus, the Vata constitution is known for an excessive amount of openness, lightness, coldness and dryness. Picture a person floating in outer space, there is no source of light or warmth within them, thus, they are attracted to sources of light and warmth – bright shiny objects, brilliant ideas, the warmth of human kindness and a nice cozy room. Likewise, emotionally they frequently may feel like they are left in the dark or are clueless about a direction in life. But when they catch some light from a star, it is as if they are in the spotlight of attention, and then they really shine. Thus, they are always looking for reassurance and guidance in how to traverse their ungrounded world. The Vatic person complains of always feeling chilled, having dry skin, or having dry, creaky joints. The slightest imbalance in his or her health or emotions will create anxiety, 'spaciness', doubt, colon troubles and insomnia. When balanced and healthy, Vatic individuals are known for their creativity, movement (dance), insightfulness and artistic talents.

The second constitution is Pitta. Here you can imagine a person full of fire. Pittic individuals are warm, energetic and have a tendency toward aggression and competition. Pitta's attributes center on the image of fire. Their digestive fire is strong, and their faces are red with the fire of circulation. Their mental radiance is often brilliant. Irritation, fevers, ulcers, oily skin and inflammatory diseases may arise when Pittas become imbalanced. These lean, muscular constitutions are known for warmth, leadership abilities, insight and vision.

The third and final constitution is Kapha, which can be pictured as a large, gentle, nurturing person. These people are strong, sturdy, and soft. Their digestion is slow and their body is cold and bulky. When they become imbalanced, there is a wetness to their illness, which may appear in the form of edema, wet sounding coughs, chronic sinus infections, and digestive problems. These people are also prone to excessive weight gain and resistance to change. Kaphas are known to be loyal, dependable, grounded and consistent. They are tremendous readers and problem solvers.

All people contain these three Ayurvedic constitutions in some proportion. For instance, I had an aunt who was 5 feet tall, weighed 230 pounds, had consistently oily skin and suffered from mild depression. Her Ayurvedic constitution was probably 90 percent Kapha, and 10 percent Pitta/Vata. Thus, she was a Kaphic person. The majority of individuals have two predominant constitutions, for example 45 percent Vata, 45 percent Pitta and 10 percent Kapha. This individual would be called a Vata-Pitta person. Some individuals also have an equal proportion of all three constitutions, approximately 33 percent Vata, 33 percent Pitta and 33 percent Kapha. This individual would be called Vata-Pitta-Kapha or VPK.

Ayurveda takes the concept of Vata, Pitta and Kapha even further. The terms Vata, Pitta, and Kapha are also applied to all preferences and activities. Thus there is "Vatic sleep," "Pittic sleep," and "Kaphic sleep." So my aunt most likely experienced Kaphic sleep due to the predominance of her Kaphic constitution. Likewise, Vata, Pitta and Kapha apply to thoughts, emotions, diseases and foods.

For example, salad is a typical Vatic food – cold, dry and uncooked. Vatic sleep is light and dreamy. Vatic activities include running and rushing. A typical Pittic food is a spicy burrito – spicy and oily. Pittic sleep is brief and restless, with a huge appetite upon awakening. Pittic activities center around intense competition. The representative

Kaphic food is ice cream – heavy, fat-filled and rich. Kaphic sleep is deep and prolonged. Kaphic activities are usually slow and require little physical effort. In later chapters we will discuss the importance of the three constitutions and their roles in your daily life.

There is no advantage to being one constitution or another. In Ayurveda, it becomes quite logical that certain professions fit better with certain constitutional types. Likewise, what you do for a living affects your body type and personality. Such observations provide valuable clues for career guidance and treatment planning. For example, a ballerina would commonly have a Vatic body, while a lineman on a football team would be predominantly Kapha. The energetic triathlon athlete would have a strong source of Pitta. These three constitutions merely reflect the nature of a person and his or her tendencies. When anyone becomes imbalanced, the problems that occur will align with the qualities of his or her constitution. However, a person of any constitution can be healthy and happy when he or she is kept in balance. Therefore, knowing your Ayurvedic constitution can greatly assist you in staying balanced by knowing what foods to eat, how to sleep, what life events could be particularly disturbing, and what exercises and activities would be best for you.

Until your constitution is in good balance, a general rule is that the foods you crave are probably not the best option for you. For instance, Vatas need warm, heavy, grounding foods but commonly crave cold leftovers and simple salads. Pittas need mild, cooling foods, but may prefer alcoholic beverages and hot, spicy foods -- pouring alcohol on a fire is always treacherous. Kaphas need light, spicy foods, but will sneak in donuts and cheesecake. Thus your Ayurvedic constitution reveals your preferences and the corresponding lifestyle choices to help you stay in balance.

A simple questionnaire can reveal your dominant constitution. On the following pages, place a "1" next to each attribute that applies to you. Then total each page. The end result will give you the pro-portion of each constitution that applies to you. For example, if you have scored 5 on the Vata page, 25 on the Pitta page, and 5 on the Kapha page, then your dominant constitution is Pitta. If you have two scores that are roughly equal and one that is less, you are prob-ably a combination of those two higher constitutions. If all three scores are nearly equal, then you are probably VPK.

Ayurvedic Quiz – Find out your nature

Questions on Vata (35)
Vata is a blending of air and space elements

Physical (13)
_____ Thin frame
_____ Prominent joints
_____ Very tall or short
__I__ Flat-chested
_____ Chilly
__/__ Dry kinky hair *not kinky*
__I__ Small dry eyes
__r__ Joint pain or joint instability
_____ Variable appetite/thirst
_____ Variable energy
_____ Crooked teeth
__I__ Dry, cold skin *(not cold)*
_____ Difficult to gain and maintain weight

Emotional Temperament (10)
__I__ Talks fast or a lot
_____ Indecisive
_____ Learns fast, but forgets
__I__ Enthusiastic, joyful
_____ Restless, active
_____ Sensitive to noise, lights
__I__ Creative, artistic
__I__ Intuitive
__I__ Easily worried and anxious

Under Stress (12)
__I__ Loses weight
__I__ Constipation
__I__ Excess gas
__I__ Restless/active
_____ Chronic pain
__I__ Light sleeper/insomnia
_____ Anxious/fearful
__I__ Drug use/abuse *(mild)*
_____ Panic attacks
__I__ Psychic
_____ Dry cracking joints
_____ Tendency to bite fingernails
_____ Pain is severe; cutting or throbbing

Your Vata Total: __15/2__

Questions on Pitta (35)
Pitta is a blending of fire and water elements

Physical (12)
__/__ Medium build
__|__ Athletic
__/__ Warm-blooded
_____ Oily, soft skin
____ Freckles
_____ Prematurely gray
_____ Straight fine hair
_____ Eyes red or yellow
__/__ Pink, pliable nails
_____ Excessive hunger
____ Excessive thirst
__|__ Muscular

Emotional Temperament (13)
_____ Words sharp/concise
__/__ Competitive
_____ Intelligent
__|__ Perceptive
_____ Keen memory
_____ Irritable/impatient
_____ Controlling
_____ Jealous
__|__ Courageous
_____ Organized/efficient
__|__ Successful
__|__ Natural born leader
_____ Overly eager and quick

Under Stress (10)
__|__ Rashes
_____ Excess sweat
__/__ Gastritis/ulcers
_____ High blood pressure
_____ Excess bleeding
_____ Eats hot spices
_____ Drinks alcohol to excess
_____ Anger/violent temper
__/__ Sleep sound/short
____ Body odor

Your Pitta Total: __16__

Questions on Kapha (35)
Kapha is the blending of earth and water elements

Physical (14)
_____ Thick, wide frame
__/__ Good stamina
__⊥__ Strong
_____ Well-lubricated joints
__⊥__ Weight in hips/thighs
_____ White, even teeth
_____ Thick lustrous hair
_____ Large eyes
_____ Slow/regular bowels
_____ Thick oily cool skin
__/__ Slow digestion
__⊥__ Difficulty losing weight
__⎮__ Gain weight easily
__/__ Large stools

Emotional Temperament (11)
_____ Slow speech
__⊥__ Calm
__⊥__ Responsible
__⎮__ Steady faith
__⎮__ Slow memory, but with good retention
__⊥__ Stubborn
__⎮__ Forgiving
__⊥__ Empathic
__⎮__ Nurturing
__⎮__ Loyal
__⎮__ Good-natured

Under Stress (10)
_____ Over sleeps
__⎮__ Overeats or loss of appetite
_____ Excess mucus
__⎮__ Water retention
__⎮__ Overweight
__⎮__ Lazy/inert
_____ Greedy
_____ Complacent
_____ Depressed
_____ Chilly

Your Kapha Total: _21_

Grand Totals — which
constitution are you?
Vata: _16_
Pitta: _14_
Kapha: _21_

Summary

Now that you know your dominant constitution(s), you can begin to understand the importance of this self-knowledge. If my dear aunt, who suffered from mild depression, had known that her Ayurvedic constitution was Kapha, she would have realized that exercise was a wonderful therapy for her. This is because Kaphas have a tendency toward inertia, and movement is therapeutic for them. However, had she been a Pitta, movement therapy and intense exercise likely would not have helped her depression. She would have needed to express herself, possibly in writing or song, so that she could let out her emotions without becoming more upset.

Each disease is also classified as Vata, Pitta or Kapha. Some diseases are primarily experienced by Kaphas, thus these diseases are called Kaphic diseases. But it is important to realize that any one of the three constitutions can become imbalanced in any person. A strongly Vatic person can develop a Pittic disorder by subjecting himself or herself to Pitta-aggravating influences (foods, exercises, etc.) This is true for all three of the constitutions, even though it is more likely that a person will develop a disease that is aligned with his or her own constitution (a Pittic person is more likely to develop a Pittic illness). Therefore, it is important for you to have an understanding of all three of the constitutions.

Now that you have a better understanding of yourself at this elemental level, you will be able to more skillfully choose the best therapies for you. Throughout this text, I will refer back to these three fundamental constitutions of Vata, Pitta and Kapha. You will come to further understand the importance of your Ayurvedic constitution in menu planning, sleeping, and exercising.

CHAPTER SUMMARY

- *To know which path will take you to happiness, you must first know who you are, what you are and what resources you have available.*

- *Understanding the three Ayurvedic constitutions will provide you with a foundation from which you can go on to understand yourself at deeper levels.*

- *When you make your choices in life with respect to your knowledge of yourself and your constitution, you will be less likely to suffer from imbalances in any area of life.*

ACTION ITEMS

- *Think of someone you know who clearly personifies each of the three Ayurvedic constitutions.*

- *Take the "Ayurvedic Quiz" to find out your constitution.*

- *Make a list of activities you engage in or foods or beverages you consume that may not be helpful for your constitution.*

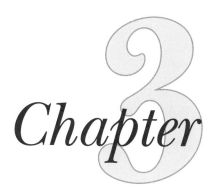

Chapter

Living with Purpose
Achieving Purpose and Clarity

INTRODUCTION

Designing and building a lifestyle to generate and maintain happiness, begins with a personal philosophy and life purpose. Knowing your basic beliefs, goals and aspirations will make traversing the path of happiness easier and more successful. In my youth I did not always know what I wanted to accomplish from day to day. I had no consistent criteria by which I could prioritize my life. How could I possibly find happiness if I did not even know myself at this basic level?

Being a writer, I have always found that putting my thoughts and ideas on paper helps give them clarity and power. When I first began to formulate a personal philosophy, I filled many tablets of paper as I tried to pin myself down. What was really important to me and why? What did I really believe about me and my life?

In the end, I realized that it is not the beliefs themselves that are important, but the understanding that I gained from my own inquiry about my life goals. Once you understand yourself and your basic operating systems, you can begin to build a foundation upon which happiness can flourish. The cornerstone to this entire process begins with the self-acceptance that is born from recognizing and respecting yourself and your life. Granted, you may not be living the life you want, but you can enjoy living the life you have. As my first college professor in education would remind us repeatedly in his country slang, "We ain't what we are gonna be, we ain't what we are supposed to be, but we ain't what we were either."

As a physician assistant and as a teacher of meditation, I have witnessed firsthand the troubles that arise from not understanding yourself and your purpose. When you do not understand yourself, or accept what you do understand, it becomes much easier to fall prey to the desires and fantasies of others.

Allow me to illustrate this point with a true story. One day a young college-aged fellow appeared at my door. I had not seen him since he was a young boy. After a few minutes of questioning, I realized the source of his distress: his own lack of self-understanding and purpose.

> *You may not be living the life you want, but you can enjoy living the life you have.*

"What would happen if you did exactly what you wanted to do?" I asked my young client. The smile on his face instantly returned—a smile that had been missing for months. It turned out that he had been tormented with conflicting messages from parents, peers, advisors and siblings. My question seemed to explode apart his torturous inner dialogue. He had put too much emphasis on the pleasing of others, never once asking himself what was best for his own personal growth. He had spent his entire life trying to please others!

For the rest of the hour, we went on to discuss what it would mean for him to be authentic, unique and living with purpose. He would have to give up his tendency to please others and start to live for himself. Right there in my office he realized that once he began doing so, his conflicts would evaporate. Over the course of the next few visits he outlined his goals and aspirations for the next five years. They had been lying unheard in his mind and heart. This simple act greatly diminished his current conflicts. His self-selected solutions immediately became clear and he left my office with newfound determination and purpose.

This story is hardly unique. So many of my patients have never clearly defined their goals. Others have defined their goals, but spend much of their time working unconsciously against them. Living with purpose means understanding yourself – your ambitions and aspirations – and living in accordance with them.

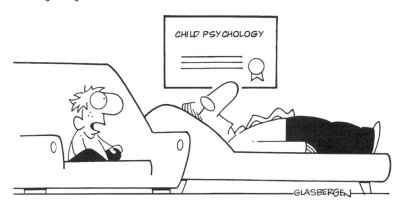

"You're spending the best years of your life doing a job that you hate so you can buy stuff you don't need to support a lifestyle you don't enjoy. Sounds crazy to me!"

You will meet three types of people in any environment. There are those who are *time-oriented* and focus their efforts around the number of hours or years that they work. There are those who are *goal-oriented* and constantly chase after the fruits of their labor. However, the happiest people always seem to be those who are *purpose-oriented*. They learn how to absorb all the blows in life as they continue to pursue the realization of their dreams. Such people develop an unlimited capacity to accept every situation and transform it into good.

Regardless of your orientation to work, passion can dominate your decisions – causing you to feel consumed by your job or mesmerized by your relationships. When left alone passion can wreak havoc. When enjoined with its companion, passion quickens your success in life. Compassion is the companion to passion. This attitude of understanding and viewing all sides of an issue will keep your actions safe and balanced. Without compassion in your efforts, your friends and family may feel distanced from your love.

To gain a better understanding of your purpose, well chosen guidelines can help you maintain this balance between passion and compassion. There are some people who become so ambitious toward their goals that they lose sight of everything else. This is not the route to happiness.

Patanjali, the codifier of the Yoga Sutras, left a blueprint for how to live with purpose. Somewhere between 250 BC and 300 AD (the exact date is widely disputed) he wrote down five principles to be considered when making important decisions. He also wrote five daily observances that can aid you in the pursuit of your purposes. Together these 10 rules and practices have helped shape people's lives for thousands of years. Only by understanding your own inner workings can you truly become happy. Otherwise you are playing a game without even knowing the rules. If you wish to be truly happy now, then in the next few pages you will be so glad that you are here.

THE FIVE PRINCIPLES OF LIVING WITH PURPOSE

PRINCIPLE ONE: DO NO HARM
(MOST IMPORTANT)

The first rule of medicine is *Primum non nocere*, which means, "In the first place, do no harm." One day, while reading the Yoga Sutras, I came across "Ahimsa" – the Sanskrit term for non-harming. It meant the very same thing that Hippocrates was implying in his Latin expression of *Primum non nocere*. I heard it, I read it and many years later, I taught it. But I had no idea it was a secret code.

It was one of those secrets so powerful that it was hidden in plain view. I thought it only meant, "do not harm the patient," but in reality, it meant something much greater. Today it is still known as the first rule of medicine, but in truth, it is the declaration of how healing occurs — if you do not harm yourself, you will never harm others. The only way we can harm ourselves is to ignore the voice of our conscience because our conscience will never let us harm ourselves or others.

This phrase protects us from actions and internal judgments that lead to guilt and shame. Today these two emotions are commonly used as teaching tools. They are a poor choice. In my own upbringing, feeling guilty and ashamed never led to a positive result.

> *The only way we can harm ourselves is to ignore the voice of our conscience.*

When Panditji first taught this principle of non-harming to me, he said, "Be nice to yourself, and be nice to others." It was immediately clear that the first goal was for me to be nice to myself. A few months later he saw me failing to do this and he then turned to me and said, "How can a human being be happy if he treats himself as his own worst enemy? What you need to do is always reward yourself; never punish yourself."

I thought about this over and over — "*only reward yourself*," even when you make a mistake? Did he speak in error? Was he supporting error over accuracy? The more I thought, the more convinced I became that it was another cryptic code – one that would unveil a major breakthrough for me, personally and professionally.

In those uncommon moments that inspire all of us, I finally cracked the code. It was a message about love. The source of non-violence is unconditional love – it is both an attitude and a touchstone. This love nurtures our compassion and corrects erroneous views that lead to self-condemnation. It is love without condition and it begins with yourself; it begins at home. Before I could unconditionally love my family, friends, and patients, I needed to unconditionally love myself, even when I was in error. There is simply no way around this truth. Indeed, this first principle is more important than the remaining four. It keeps you safe and keeps the world safe. According to the yogic texts, when you become firmly established in kindness — which is what "doing no harm" means — other people who come near you will naturally lose any feelings of hostility. Once I understood this first principle, I saw how many of my patients were failing to abide by it.

Ralph was in his sixties and wanted to mend his relationship with his son and daughter. A gambler and alcoholic for most of his life, he lost his children to a divorce and a sea of whiskey. Sobriety came late in life and birthed a new man. He was not able to locate his children for several of his new sober years. During that time, he lived in Los Angeles and started practicing yoga. His body was not able to move into the stretching poses that the posters displayed at the studio, but his teacher inspired him to read about the philosophy of yoga. In doing so he learned about non-violence, the first and most important rule to follow.

As Ralph started being kind to himself, he felt conflicted. He did not deny his mistakes from the past, but the memories of days gone by made him feel hypocritical. How could he be kind to himself when he still felt he deserved to be punished?

Through the magic of the Internet, he found my Web site, and we started corresponding by phone and email. He was naturally philosophical and an avid reader of my online newsletters. It was the inspiration of ancient stories about overcoming guilt and shame that gave him hope of triumph. But it was his intellect that brought his attention to his past mistakes, even though his best intentions were to move forward.

My conversations with Ralph turned to the topic of non-violence. Ralph did not realize that his habit of self-condemnation was in conflict with his beliefs about non-violence. His intellect was actually causing harm to himself every time he recalled an unpleasant event that led him to feel regret or remorse. He was mentally "beating himself up" and I helped him realize that it had to stop. Because of his philosophical nature, I knew that when he heard the ancient story of Jaigishavya's struggle with the same issue, he could then apply the same methodology to uproot his own misery.

Jaigishavya was a sincere yogi trying to break free of his old habit patterns. He became entrapped by his own intellect and sought the counsel of the sage Avatya. This gentle sage advised him to sharpen his intellect so that he could understand his infatuation with the errors of his past. He explained, "Your interest in your past is an indication of your desire to reclaim it. And this desire to reclaim the past is due to your attachment. You are aware that most of your past is painful. Logically, you should have no desire to re-associate yourself with painful events, yet you are drawn to them. Why? It is because you are attached to your actions, the fruit of your actions and their subtle impressions. You treasure them in your mind, although you know how useless, ugly and painful they are."

WHY WE KEEP THINKING ABOUT PAINFUL THINGS

Most of us are accustomed to the idea of attachment to pleasurable objects and experiences and yet we commonly dwell on our mistakes more than our successes. Yoga and modern biochemistry discuss how the comfort of familiar habits may be stronger than the usefulness of the habit. This familiarity keeps us recalling and repeating unhelpful activities and unwanted impulses. The misery of perpetually doing that which we no longer wish to do, and yet feel helpless to stop, is brought to a halt through non-attachment.

"When a memory upsets you or thrills you, it is your attachment giving energy to your past. You can instantly neutralize the past with the power of non-attachment," advised the sage.

Ralph, like Jaigishavya, was drawn toward painful and disappointing memories of his past and yet the same images also engendered a sense of pleasure. The pleasure came from the comfort of something familiar, even though it was painful. The concern here was that Ralph's attachment to such recollections might motivate him to act out the past again.

"Attachment," explained Avatya, "is like the nutrients a seed needs in order to sprout. Once you no longer provide these nutrients, the seeds of the past will lose their capacity to grow into destiny."[3]

Ralph started to practice non-violence toward himself by loosening his fascination with the errors of his past. Over several months, he observed and corrected every instance where his intellect attempted to harm his emotions and ruin his self-esteem and confidence. Every time his unwanted memories of gambling or alcoholism came into his awareness, he redoubled his efforts toward being kind to himself.

It was definitely not an easy task. No matter how many times his mind reminded him of his past faults, he continued to unconditionally love and accept himself.

Finally, the day came when he was reunited with his children — an event that, while desired, he had also dreaded for many years. Ralph's tale about his wonderful reunion and his children's acceptance of their long-lost father made him one of my favorite teachers of kindness. That kindness brought healing to years of confusion and hurt. I will always remember Ralph as a symbol of non-violence in action.

> *When you treat yourself with kindness, then you will naturally treat others with kindness.*

This first principle of self-transformation, non-violence, must begin with yourself. When you treat yourself with kindness, then you will naturally treat others with kindness. This was the lesson Panditji was teaching when he said, "Always reward yourself, never punish." Without weighing your merits and demerits, learn to find ways to make friends with your mind so that you only reward yourself and never punish yourself and you will have mastered this first principle.

SUMMARY:

- *In the practice of non-violence, the most important component and essential starting point is non-violence toward yourself. Never condemn, criticize or punish yourself.*

ACTION ITEM:

- *Practice rewarding yourself and actively engaging in not criticizing yourself.*

Principle Two: Truthfulness

Truthfulness is the second principle of living with purpose. Truthfulness lightens your burdens, boosts your spirits, and brings about the insights for a peaceful resolution. Truth is always inspiring, clarifying and immediately useful.

If being honest or truthful is violent to ourselves or to others, then it is not the truthfulness that the ancient sages described. Truth is always spoken in a way that quickens your journey to the goal of life. The "honest facts" are like readouts of technical data. They are barren facts not meant to contain any judgment or opinion. We commonly encounter such honesty when viewing the ledgers of our bank account or the instruction manual that helps us assemble our new bookcase. When the ancient sages were teaching the concept of truthfulness, the value of kindness and the self-esteem of all parties involved were placed above hurtful honesty. In building and maintaining relationships, use the principle of truthfulness that is filled with love.

I experimented with these two different viewpoints of truthfulness over and over. Sometimes they flowed smoothly in my life and at other times they were in harsh opposition to one another. As a medical practitioner, I had to learn how to share the glaring results of a blood test in the most compassionate manner. When duty called me to be the bearer of bad news to my patients, my mind and my heart relied heavily on these first two principles of non-violence and truthfulness. As you experiment with them in your life, eventually you will find gentleness in your thought and speech that will allow you to deliver honest data in the most kind and caring manner.

Summary:

- *Truthfulness is valuable, but only so long as it is not violent to ourselves or to others. Truthfulness must be skillfully practiced along with the principle of non-violence, which always comes first.*

Action Items:

- *Before speaking or acting, think beyond your truthfulness and consider whether or not you are also being loving and compassionate.*

Principle Three: Abstain From All Forms of Theft

The third principle of living with purpose is abstaining from all forms of theft. It is a sign of true self-reliance when all forms of stealing vanish from your mind. The joy of unconditional love and honesty will build your self-esteem to the point that the idea of needing something from someone else in order to be happy becomes ludicrous. Thoughts of shoplifting, plagiarism, and seducing the affection of others completely disappear from your awareness.

When you realize that the possessions of others — physical and non-physical — neither fulfill nor threaten your happiness or perfection, then you have attained mastery over this third principle. With this mastery also comes the source of true wealth. The ancient yoga texts strongly emphasize the importance of non-stealing. They say that as long as we have the tendency to misuse or clutch things that are not ours, we remain ordinary and abide by the regular rules of nature. But when we rise above these tendencies, we gain freedom from the ordinary rules of life. The greatest wealth we can attain is a happy mind and a healthy body. The ancient texts declare that true wealth kisses the feet of those who no longer desperately misuse, hoard or grasp the objects of the world.

Swami Rama used a bottle of shampoo to teach me this principle. Karen and I had the habit of bringing home shampoo bottles from hotels with the goal of donating them to our local women's shelter. Over time, my generosity spread further than the bounds of the local shelter as I started to maintain a small collection of shampoo in my suitcase. Instead of giving the bottles away, I started secretly hoarding a small bounty for no known reason. At some level I was afraid that the next hotel would not supply enough cleanser for my balding head. What woke me up was Swamiji's comment about how hoarding anything at the personal level maintains the myth of scarcity. He spoke of trusting that what you need will be there – this can become a self-fulfilling prophecy. It creates an attraction to solutions and discourages worry from entering your mind. His words had caught me red-handed, and with a blushed-face my behavior instantly changed. This tiny adjustment in my hotel etiquette drastically decreased my newly-discovered feelings of vulnerability and scarcity. Until Swamiji pointed this out to me, my behaviors were subconscious and unfounded. No longer feeling fearful of shortages on my journey through life has increased my sense of trust in the world and the trust that what I need will be provided. I have never been disappointed.

> *True wealth kisses the feet of those who no longer desperately misuse, hoard, or grasp the objects of the world.*

SUMMARY:

- *The principle of abstaining from theft is attained naturally when one realizes that "the possessions of others – physical and non-physical – can neither fulfill nor threaten your happiness."*

ACTION ITEMS:

- *Examine your life for things which are not yours, but which you cling to or desire nonetheless. Acknowledge that they do not belong to you and let go of your attachment to them.*

PRINCIPLE FOUR: MOVING THROUGH THE WORLD WITH A UNIFIED MIND

A unified mind is the antithesis of a scattered and divided mind. When your mind becomes the employee of your conscience, then your mind no longer harbors fantasies of fear and attack. Grooming your mind to listen to your conscience is one of the main themes of this book. This achievement is possible for everyone, and once this union is established, wherever you travel in the world you will feel an inner sense of unity with all people and places. The experience has been described as walking with a constant awareness of a divine presence or highest virtue. To observe such an inward phenomena implies a continence or self-mastery of the sensory network that feeds your mind, as well as a personal philosophy of unconditional acceptance or love.

According to yoga science, the senses reach outward and contact their chosen object and then bring the image and experience of that object back into the mind. The experiences that are more exciting and stimulating create a much larger impact on your mind, thus shifting your mood in a major fashion. But their impact can be much longer lasting than a passing mood.

The reverberations of powerful stimuli become the foundation for the development of our subtle habits and interests. Thus, we see people who are driven by their taste for sweets, others who crave touch, and some who crave music and conversation. The sexual urge is the most powerful and, therefore, can become the most disruptive if not directed and channeled properly.

Intense cravings drain a great deal of energy from both your mind and body. If you allow your mind and body to become weakened by these cravings, you may lose some of the strength you need to withstand the challenges of disease, old age, and death. The science and psychology of yoga offer us the insights to understand this phenomena and the methodology for self-transformation.

The most practical apparatus to change the quality of the mind is the transportation of data through the five senses and the buddhi as discussed in Chapter One. When unsupervised, the senses run out into the world and make contact with a multitude of objects. Immediately upon contact, the senses flood the mind with the impressions and power of their experience. If the senses continue to do this in a random fashion, the contents and interests of the mind may become unmanageable. Thus, this fourth principle of learning how to move through the world in a unified manner requires that you learn how to understand and control your senses as well as your sensual urges.

> *The more you become free from the intensity of sensory cravings, the greater your joy and clarity will become.*

For example, sometimes I have the craving for a cookie. However, once I eat the cookie, I may immediately want another one. It is the nature of desire that fulfilling a craving often does not bring it to an end. This is also true for stronger desires. Therefore, learn to live in moderation and fully understand that fulfilling your desires will not end your desires altogether. This implies the ability to understand and direct your choices of desire and activity. The more you become free from the intensity of sensory cravings, the greater your joy and clarity will become. Refraining from the fulfillment of all desires is not the goal. The goal is to control the senses in order to achieve deeper levels of inner awareness. Without a comprehensive understanding, any pro-hibition of desire commonly leads to an imbalance in both food and sleep. Thus, all desires must be studied, understood and mastered.

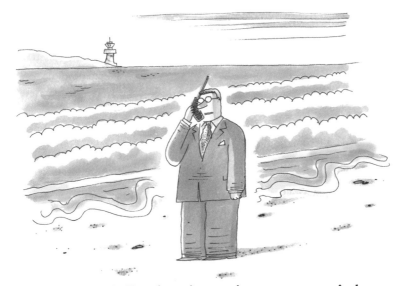

"Not much, Frank . . . just trying to get my mind around this 'vacation' concept."

Any observer of their own mind or humanity, at any scale, can readily see the impulsiveness of our behavior. When spontaneous im-pulses or everyday desires are fulfilled without merit, chaos can domi-nate our lives. When Patanjali wrote this fourth principle, he gave us a vision of how a happy mind moves through the day – unified, sat-isfied and inspired. He acknowledged the multitude of distractions and desires that would quickly make anyone forget their bond with humanity. This fourth principle of self-mastery teaches and models the manners of channeling and choosing our sensual urges with dig-nity and virtue.

When desires build to the point of preoccupation — whether they are real or imaginary – then that desire dominates your life. You must have the freedom of choice to direct your attention in an appropriate and timely manner before an unwanted buildup occurs. Mastery of any urge requires a very broad understanding of your personality and habits. Gaining mastery of your sensuality implies understanding and choice – it is not a path of suppression or denial. As you begin to explore the human within you, it may seem that your inward-dwelling happiness is weaker than the objects of desire embedded in your sensory impressions. Do not worry. This tendency to instantly embrace impulses can be monitored and transformed. Every chapter of this book will provide you with a different strategy to lessen the strength of unwanted impulses. Logic is no match for a powerful urge. You will learn how to align your diet, breathing patterns, exercise, etc. in a manner that supports your logic and goals.

Start with simple urges that you feel you can successfully transform, and then move forward to deeper issues as your confidence increases. In time, you will be able to guide your awareness to look within. Then you will see and experience that true joy is more powerful and more desirable than the urges of your past. With this system, you transform your tendencies gradually; there is no need to fight with them.

I heard a cocaine addict describe his life as one who sets his own hair on fire and then tries to beat out the flames with an iron skillet. The blind actions of sensuality can drag the kindest person into a cesspool of confusion and regret. This draining of your sanity and joy can ruin your health and your life. Likewise, control is also the means for re-gaining and rejuvenating the vitality of your body, breath and mind.

If your desire for the taste of a donut or the smell of a good cigar is mandatory in your life, then learning to control your senses can reduce these activities to simple options instead of carved-in-stone mandates. All of us can imagine the drain of constantly being battered by urges we wish we could control. The failure of every diet, weight loss program, and exercise regimen can be traced back to answering desires that are oppositional to our healthier goals.

Mastering your desires will bring you great freedom and contentment every moment of the day. The ancient texts say that enthusiasm
and courage come from feeling free to choose how you live your life.
The key is in understanding your desires, deciding which to ignore
and which to fulfill, with the overarching goal of attaining unshak-
able happiness. You will master your desires and find the freedom
you seek when you do not suppress and do not indulge.

Summary:

- *Learning to control your senses and gently guiding them to engage in
  constructive and helpful activities will allow you to begin obtaining
  freedom from the intensity of sensory cravings. In their place, you
  will begin to experience your inward-dwelling joy.*

Action Items:

- *In order to practice the concept of "do not suppress and do not indulge," the next time you desire something which is not helpful for
  you, say to yourself: "That's all right for my mind to desire that object, but I have control over my body and I will not go and get that
  object for my mind."*

Principle Five: Freedom from Possessiveness

The fifth principle of living with purpose is freedom from possessiveness. This freedom is multi-layered: you become free of the gross addic-
tions and dependencies on material objects and, at a much deeper level,
you become free of labeling yourself and others. We either proudly
display or hide from every label, diagnosis, or title that we acquire in
life. In order to attain this fifth principle, it is necessary to transcend all
forms of gathering objects and labels -- external and internal.

The principle of "non-possessiveness" has two aspects: a worldly part and a personal identity part. Everyone has an aunt or uncle who is a packrat, constantly gathering every small trinket from the world. The first aspect of non-possessiveness involves reducing your attachment to worldly goods that may hinder your journey to joy.

The second aspect is the way we "possess" our identity. Some people are very attached to their identity as a bodybuilder, a sports car owner, or a millionaire. This kind of possessiveness can also limit your happiness.

The secret to mastering the principle of non-possessiveness is to perfect the art of non-acceptance. This means that you no longer accept anything that delays or detours your journey. Non-possessiveness means not letting the people and objects in your life possess you. In non-acceptance, it is perfectly fine to have worldly possessions as long as they do not hinder your happiness. It is wonderful to be the CEO of a Fortune 500 company as long as it brings joy and not misery. This is the art of non-acceptance.

Non-acceptance is a practical approach to living your life. When your happiness is reliant on the physical objects of the world, it is subject to decay and destruction. All objects can break or be taken; this is why happiness must be found within. Therefore, you can learn to recognize the objects that limit your ability to find inner happiness and choose better options. One such example is a plasma-screen television. For some of my patients, if I gave them a new plasma television, they would never accomplish any contemplation, meditation, reading, or self-study. Instead, they would spend their entire free time in front of the television. For these patients, a plasma television would definitely hinder their progress toward happiness. In the spirit of non-acceptance, sometimes you must reject material objects.

Non-acceptance also offers some solutions for overcoming issues of identity and labeling. Any label or identity that does not enhance your self-respect or self-development should be ignored. In my first book, *Happiness: The Real Medicine,* I briefly discussed my childhood identity of being a mistake-maker. A seemingly harmless joke and a teacher's label changed my childhood for the worse. Years later, I now fully understand the power and damage labeling can cause. Do not label yourself and do not label others.

> *When your happiness is reliant on the physical objects of the world, it is subject to decay and destruction.*

Frank, one of my dearest patients, came to me with terrible news. He had suffered a brain stem injury due to a fall at work and the doctor's prognosis was not good. In fact, the doctors told him that he had an irreversible condition causing his brain to be imbalanced. Frank was devastated and frightened. Ever since his accident he had migraines, changing moods and strange food allergies that caused him to lose almost all of his body fat. At the brink of hopelessness, he came to my doorstep.

For almost two years he had been slowly deteriorating mentally and physically. His diet had become so restricted, due to his allergies, that he was only eating fish. When I began to discuss his prognosis with him, he was very grim and gloomy. I immediately realized exactly what had happened and his next year of office visits with me proved it to be true.

Frank had become a victim of his own diagnosis to the extent that he believed his physician despite the fact that his physician could not pinpoint his exact condition. Even after I treated him homeopathically and his allergies and migraines were cured, he still believed that his brain was not functioning and that he was doomed. His mind could simply not accept the fact that he was steadily improving. Slowly, over the course of many months, his experience and our discussions fostered the idea of being completely healthy again.

There is an old joke in medicine that says, "What do you do when your doctor tells you that you have three weeks to live?" The answer is, "Get another doctor." To search for other options and insights is not to disregard the first doctor. But in the search for happiness, the principle of non-acceptance teaches you to only accept that information which is helpful to your self-growth and self-esteem.

In Frank's case, he needed to get another opinion and he needed to have someone tell him that healing was a possibility. Instead, he had completely changed his identity into being this fellow with an incurable disease. Years later, Frank slowly shifted his identity and his behavior back to being a healthy individual. His healing continues today.

Once you have a firm understanding of the principle of non-acceptance, then non-possessiveness is easy and comes naturally. You will no longer accept anything that can threaten your happiness and wholeness. At this stage of understanding, you cannot be bribed by

> *Any label or identity that does not enhance your self-respect or self-development should be ignored.*

charms or promises because you know what is helpful for your own self-development. Remember that non-possessiveness does not mean giving away all your worldly goods and living in poverty. It means not becoming overly infatuated with the objects of the world and your self identity. Everything in this world is here for you to use. But use it graciously as a guest — don't clutch it desperately like a beggar.

Comfort comes first as a guest,
Then becomes your host,
And eventually your master.
It is best to keep comfort as a guest.
-Unknown

SUMMARY:

- *Becoming dependent upon either physical objects in the world or any identity that you have constructed for yourself will not improve your ability to find happiness, it will limit it.*

ACTION ITEMS:

- *Contemplate what you consider to be your identity and your possessions, and then contemplate what would be left if you had none of those objects or ideas.*

THE FIVE DAILY OBSERVANCES FOR LIVING WITH PURPOSE

Swami Rama taught that "discipline is doing that which creates the highest joy." To diminish stress in your life, self-discipline must be imposed from the inside. This sort of discipline is only for those who understand it and choose it for themselves. Swamiji reminded all of us that "no" should only be spoken to ourselves and not to others. It is we who must guide and monitor our choices in life.

The five principles discussed in the following section form the best foundation for character development and self-reliance. This explanation of these daily observances will allow you to see the power of these concepts and the most common misapplications of such great insights.

CLEANLINESS

Cleanliness refers to your body, breath, mind and relationships. It is the active process of diminishing all impurities including junk, clutter, falsehoods and annoyances. It is not a state of arrogance and superiority, but rather a frank recognition that there can be endless worldly diversions from the goal of happiness. When you recognize your own purity, you begin to make choices that support your new identity, both inwardly and outwardly. When you begin to live your life in a manner that maintains your purity, you become filled with a sense of contentment.

Sometimes indecision creates clutter in the mind and soon this inner hesitation manifests itself as physical clutter in your office, basement, garage or attic as possessions begin to pile up. Desktops and countertops can disappear into an array of correspondence, bills and junk mail. The solution is a quick response to every moment and event. Modern life rarely provides you the luxury to delay your reactions to your family and your world. As you understand yourself and your relationship with the world, you will begin to make better decisions for yourself. This is cleanliness in action. Removing physical clutter can help you think more clearly and promote an inner cleanliness.

Meditation and contemplation become the tools that remove emotional and mental clutter. You transition from the yard and garage, to the desk and the countertops, and finally find moments to spend quieting the mental chatter within. As you incorporate regularity into cleaning both your inner and outer world, then life becomes much easier at every level. Gradually these habits will help reveal your true identity, bringing joy, gladness and mirth in its wake.

My office will occasionally present me with a patient who has taken the observance of cleanliness to the extremes of social and psychological dysfunction. For several years I had a steady flow of such overly-enthusiastic purists. You have probably heard of or met someone like Jill.

Jill was a cheerleader when she was in high school and always strived to be an exemplary model in school and sports. After college and a wholesome marriage, she thought she was on the fast track to a good life. One day at the local bookstore, she was in an absentminded rush and forgot to pay for a book in her hand. Caught in the parking lot by a security guard, Jill was mortified. Her shock and spurious ramblings almost convinced the store owner that she had done it on purpose. When her husband arrived and calmed her down, the matter was quickly resolved and her mere absentmindedness was revealed. But for Jill, she had irreparably stained her good name.

It took several weeks for her husband to notice the extreme cleanliness of the house. Jill had started to constantly straighten and organize their home. Dusting, vacuuming, and rearranging the furniture became her full-time obsession. Unconsciously she was seeking a way to purify herself and her environment in hopes that the stain of humiliation would vanish from her thoughts. Fortunately, she was brought to my office soon after these behaviors began. In this early stage, she was still only focused on cleaning her home and had not developed further obsessions with germs and her own body's purity.

Upon completing my initial interview with Jill, I prescribed a homeopathic remedy known to resolve such obsessive-compulsive behavior. Within days, Jill's extreme behaviors resolved and her self-esteem was regained. In later discussions, I helped normalize her actions by explaining how purity is a common means in starting the path of self-transformation.

The most common misunderstanding of purity that I see professionally is in regard to diet. With the help of movies like *Super Size Me**, the proliferation of vegetarian and vegan cookbooks, and the unwavering medical benefits of the vegetarian diet, more and more people are seeking guidance on how to transition to vegetarianism. In seeking this guidance it is important to look for sources that provide practical and balanced advice. A vegetarian diet has many benefits, but like any other diet it is best implemented in a manner that ensures proper nutrient and energy intake. When trying to purify one's diet, it is easy to become overzealous to the point where changes that were meant to promote health become detrimental. Expert counsel and extreme caution must be taken, including medical supervision, before engaging in long-term fasting or a minimalist's diet with a severely reduced food intake. Alex was a patient of mine who became a perfect example of the dangers of fasting.

Alex was a single man who became a devotee of a self-proclaimed and well-published spiritual guide. After attending a retreat in Cali-

---

* *Super Size Me is a multiple award-winning documentary. The producer of the film, Morgan Spurlock, subjected himself to eating only McDonald's food for 30 days. The physiological damage Spurlock suffered during the 30 days of filming was astounding. Furthermore, references throughout the film to the political and financial domination and expenditures of fast food companies makes for a very eye-opening and educational experience.*

fornia with this celebrity, Alex became a pure vegetarian. The problem was that he became such a pure vegetarian that he limited his diet to the point that he was starving himself. He lost drastic amounts of weight, sold his car (to help prevent global warming) and was finally found completely disoriented while wandering the streets of a small California town. He had never made it back to the Midwest after his week-long retreat. His parents flew him home and a psychiatrist in my office started him on an anti-psychotic medication. One day I saw this thin shell of a man in the hallway at work and I pulled him aside.

Alex told me what had happened. He had a clear Vatic** disruption caused by severe weight loss and fasting. He would need to quickly regain some weight in order to become mentally and emotionally balanced. I consulted with his psychiatrist and we began a food program for Alex. I made sure that my plan was nutritious and honored Alex's preference for vegetarian food, but the important part was just to get him eating again.

> *Mental purity manifests in the form of determination, compassion and happiness.*

It took almost nine weeks for the old, reliable Alex to reemerge. Pleased with his weight gain and sensibility, his psychiatrist was happy to gradually eliminate all of his medications. Alex's desire to be pure was well-intentioned, but lacked the personal guidance that he needed.

Purity and cleanliness start on the physical level and yield many

---

** *A "Vatic" disruption is an Ayurvedic term for an imbalanced physiology caused, in this case, by fasting and extreme weight loss. Such conditions can cause one to become ungrounded and mentally imbalanced. Their 'spaciness' and non-attachment is not spiritual attainment, it is pathology that needs treatment.*

health benefits. While this is easy to achieve, it is also important to be practical in your approach to purity and avoid extremes that drain your emotions and disrupt your concentration. A positive attitude and proper discrimination will help keep your mind clear and clean. Mental purity manifests in the form of determination, compassion and happiness. In my experience, once your diet is simple and clean, then yogic breathing exercises (called pranayamas) and meditation are the most immediate means to purifying the mind. I will discuss them both in future chapters.

SUMMARY:

- *When you recognize your own inner purity, you will begin to make decisions in life that support and maintain that purity in an internal and external sense.*

ACTION ITEMS:

- *Pick something simple (make a small healthy change in your diet, try a pranayama exercise, clean a part of your living space that is typically cluttered, etc...) to add a little cleanliness to your life. Observe the effect it has on you.*

CONTENTMENT

Contentment is a state whereby your inner equilibrium is balanced and calm. When you have achieved a sense of contentment, then you have also mastered stress management. Your inner calm cannot be threatened by external bustle.

The constant changes in the world present the first challenge to achieving contentment. As you fortify your senses—as we discussed in an earlier chapter — you increase your ability to maintain contentment. However, your own desires, memories and fascinations can also disturb your level of contentment. Contentment is not a passive state, but rather the result of prolonged and consistent self-discipline where you consciously *choose* to be content— regardless of the state of the world outside you and the state of the world inside you. Mind can continue to dwell on its fancies while you direct your attention higher. Like a beautiful lotus flower blossoming in muddy waters, rise above, remain above.

A lack of self-understanding creates the illusion of an inner poverty that robs our sense of contentment. Openly sharing your wealth of knowledge, love or possessions dispels this illusion and cures that inner void. Your inspiration and enthusiasm is directly proportional to the amount of charity you give in any form. Your sense of contentment blossoms with selfless and charitable deeds.

> *Your sense of contentment blossoms with selfless and charitable deeds.*

True contentment is the goal of all self-training, resulting in a state in which you are finally free from the push and pull of all desires. This achievement spawns the essential delight of living, allowing it to shine forth for the benefit of all.

SUMMARY:

- *Contentment requires you to actively choose to be content — regardless of your circumstances.*

ACTION ITEMS:

- *Practice being content in a situation in which you would not normally feel content.*

SELF-EFFORT

It is natural to want everything in life to come to you with little or no effort. However, this is rarely the case. In this book you are now learning new ideas and strategies to help you feel happier and become healthier. However, it is the amount of self-effort that you put forth that will determine your ultimate success. Changing longstanding habits and lifestyle issues will sometimes require a tremendous amount of effort on your part. Luckily, the tiniest steps in the right direction yield immediate benefits. This makes it easy for you to be inspired to make larger strides later.

The techniques are simple, practical and straightforward. I want you to be successful. The most simple and powerful way to become free of unwanted habits is to train the senses of your body with your breath. (I will share with you techniques for working with your breath in Chapter 7.) Staying on task will be difficult as long as you allow your senses to reach out and gather the delights of the day. To train the senses using your intellect alone is to create a never-ending battle between desire and reason. For centuries, yoga science has demonstrated the ease of using the breath to gain mastery and comfort in life.

With proper guidance and inspiration, you can start with a minimal amount of effort and notice that you are feeling happier. Once you have experienced this success, you will be more inspired to overcome the bigger obstacles that unveil even greater joys. Self-effort, when channeled in the correct direction, can trounce the worst habits and personality traits.

SUMMARY:

- *Even a small amount of self-effort, when sincere and in the right direction, will always yield results and can inspire you to make greater efforts to achieve greater results.*

Action Items:

- *Choose a simple point of guidance from this book and make an effort to practice it in your life, and observe the results.*

Self-Study

Self-study is the foundation upon which you can build your happiness. Carefully examine and study the aspects of your life that amplify your joy. Reminding yourself of your failures and apparent obstacles may become more disheartening than helpful, thus, focus on what *does* work for you. In the chapter on contemplation, I will fully explain the importance and power of self-study.

In my own personal quest, I always viewed my search for happiness as a journey. Any well-seasoned traveler will tell you that the most important things to have are a good map, a good guide, and insights from other travelers who have already made the journey. Self-study means acquiring knowledge that is helpful for you and learning the principles and practices that are specifically useful for you. Many people want to be "successful" or "spiritual" without a clear definition of those terms. They want it, but they aren't really sure what it is. This lack of clarity and honesty about the journey commonly leads to failure and frustration. It also can make you gullible to falling prey to false teachers who will rob you of your money or, even worse, your self-reliance. A beginning sojourner needs to follow the threefold path of self-study.

First, get to know yourself and your immediate strengths and weaknesses. Compare your self-inventory with the requirements of the journey on which you wish to embark – for me this was a journey to happiness. Study the map, find a good guide, and talk to those who have already accomplished the journey.

As you come to know your own personal needs and goals, it is then important to carefully select the resources that can help you attain your goal. I have found it to be very important to choose books, teachers and therapists that are compatible with helping me overcome my immediate hurdles. I have gone through a progression of highly-valued mentors and techniques in this process. My allegiance was not to a particular person or culture, rather it was to freedom itself. As a child, I greatly respected my first-grade teacher but 12 months after meeting her I was eager to study with my second-grade teacher. It is with this same attitude that I have studied medicine, sought counsel in the form of a personal trainer and found great benefit from fellowship. Each activity helped me understand and resolve obstacles in my journey. Incorporate the teachings and counsel of others, but allow your conscience to be your chief guide. At that point self-study can truly lead to wondrous self-transformation.

The second phase is creating time in your day or week for self-reflection where you can digest the facts and possibilities of your experiences. Sit down and think about what has happened. In the beginning I could only find time for this on the weekends. None of us wants to make the process of self-transformation overly tiresome and time-consuming. So choose a time and place that works for you.

Gradually you will see that insights and guidance, that will help you reach your goals, occur every day. And, more importantly, your self-reflection strengthens your determination as you learn to view all life events as lessons and feedback. Then you will value the wisdom gained from failure or loss. This allows you to become more realistic about your timetables and more skillful in your actions.

The third phase is the momentum birthed by the accumulation of insights gained from your self-study. A few minutes each day can build into the groundswell of insights leading to a big "aha." When you get stuck in really difficult situations on your journey, trust your past efforts to come forward with an escape plan. The accumulation of your past efforts have created a forward moving momentum that will carry you through moments of weakness or despair. No matter what, you will complete your journey.

Summary:

- *Self-study is your opportunity to take something home from the classroom of life experiences. Examine your experiences in life in combination with guidance from books, teachers and therapists to gain insights and guidance to help you toward your goals.*

Action Items:

- *Set aside a practical, realistic amount of quiet time for regular self-study.*

Spiritual Clarity – The End of Selfishness

As you become fully established in the truth of your experiential identity, you feel and realize that the ever-flowing knowledge and peace within you is the only solution to all stress and challenge. You will start to experience this constant stream of compassion as you use relaxation exercises, meditation and contemplation to loosen your grip on the objects and identities that once seemed to be essential to your life. Your vision will become broader as you open yourself to new and larger horizons. The experiences you gain from these inward practices will lead you to the source of true happiness – known to some as a spiritual or inner awakening. Yoga refers to this as Samadhi.

Pandit Rajmani explains, "The moment one realizes why the air provides oxygen to all, why the rain moistens the earth, and why the sun gives light and heat, then he feels the overflowing love and compassion of the Divine." Likewise, other commentators have defined this source, this perennial wisdom, as the ultimate reality and the origin of divine ecstasy.

Spiritual clarity is obtained as self-centered actions and decisions diminish. Some call this process "surrendering to God" or "surrendering to a higher power." This is a major switch from how our life begins. In the beginning, life is all about you. I call it the "me, me, me" phase. That's how everyone starts life. As you grow up through your infant years, you soon realized that there are other people in the world, and that they are your competition. Spiritually, this is the "It's me or you" phase. In this phase you try to out-best others in any manner. Later, you discover that working in cooperation with others could double or triple your success. This phase is called the "Me and you" phase. Commonly I see people who live in one of these first three phases and find great comfort there. While it may seem rare, everyone eventually goes beyond these first three stages to a fourth level of "I and I." This is the stage where one sees more similarities than differences between individuals, peoples and nations. Eventually the "I and I" phase concludes with a feeling that we are all interconnected. It is the classic experience of a universal oneness.

At this highest point of self-realization, you have recognized the equalities of all people, and that the entire field of life, in all its forms, constitutes a single living entity. This is an amazing and transforming insight – it is the basis of a global mind that wants to help all inhabitants of the planet. However, this realization alone is not enough to shake off your personal prejudices that arise from the historical training of your own mind, family, profession, culture and theology. As you become a global citizen, your actions and values start to reflect a more global viewpoint. Nature celebrates every moment in which one individual recognizes that their identity is inextricably enjoined with the whole of humanity. Likewise, when the river flows into the ocean, both benefit from that union. To have such an oceanic mind is to develop a universal view that evolves into the unconditional compassion of the highest love.

The evolution to this final phase is slow but constant. As you meet people of different ages, religions and cultures you realize that you have differences. Thus, your level of understanding must expand. Over time, you will no longer identify yourself by various titles that encase a limited set of options and ideas, consequently freeing you from your apparent differences with others. This transition may happen like this…

First your name and title become unimportant. When this happens, you no longer need to be known by your college credentials or professional titles. Later, your need to be ruled by your gender will become unimportant and unnecessary. This creates a domino-like effect. Once your gender no longer matters, very quickly your profession, your marital status and your age will no longer be icons defining your social identity. Freedom from these labels allows your mind to access a broader range of insight and understanding. It creates a drastic shift for the better in your ability to listen and counsel.

> *A universal view evolves into the unconditional compassion of the highest love.*

Gradually over the years, the city, state and national identities will also fall away. You become a global citizen with no prejudice against lands that did not birth you. Finally, your understanding outgrows the farthest reaches of your own philosophy and theology. Your mind beckons to enter that great void that is ever-rich with joy and wisdom.

Your conscience over time will no longer be confined to the inherent self-centeredness of ordinary life. You will continually feel a gradual joining and unification with everyone and everything. The ancient texts declare that this will become a natural, voluntary state and is the permanent residence of the wise.

Every valid spiritual text proclaims that profound meditation upon the purest form of purity will give you access to a spiritual state that some call universal oneness, enlightenment, or nirvana. These terms may blur the merit of this experience. The importance lies in broadening your life views until no one is excluded from your understanding. Selfishness has gone through a metamorphosis and births the true spirit of fellowship and communion. This experiential transformation answers every query that the ego and intellect face when sincerely considering the possibility and the nature of the divine.

> *While I have never met a supreme being, I feel it is good to imitate his or her traits of compassion, love, truth and knowledge.*

While I have never met a supreme being, I feel it is good to imitate his or her traits of compassion, love, truth, and knowledge. This inspired me to free myself of any personal history and cultural dogma that made me feel that others were in some way different from myself. This difference, whether it was elevating or degrading, was still separating. To love all, and exclude none is the goal.

Chapter Summary:

- *At this highest point of self-realization, you have recognized the equalities of all people, and that the entire field of life, in all of its forms, constitutes a single being.*

Action Items:

- *In order to evolve beyond personal prejudices, practice observing the similarities between you and people whom you previously thought of as different from you.*

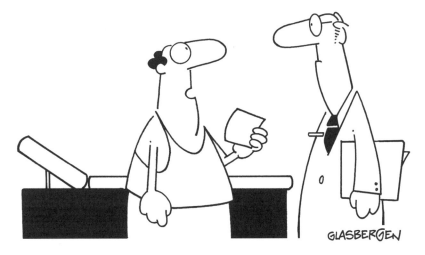

"Which 'sensible diet' do you want me to follow?
I found 123,942 of them on the internet!"

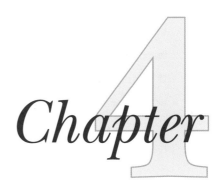

Chapter 4

The Happiness Diet

People are fascinated with food. From diet books to cookbooks, everyone wants to know how to eat more, eat less or dine like royalty. Most food-oriented literature emphasizes health benefits and social celebrations, but misses the connection between happiness and food, where food can become a conduit for good mental health and the betterment of relationships.

My goal is not to replace all that has been written on food, but simply to help you understand how food affects your mood and your experiences throughout your day. A few basic principles on how and what to eat will guide you toward the quality of life you are seeking.

- Foods can determine your moods. If you keep eating the same way, you will keep feeling the same way. In the next few pages, I will show you how food can affect your emotions.

> *Your garden and your shopping cart can replace your psychologist and your internist and help to solve global starvation.*

- Foods can kill you. Most diseases and deaths can be attributed either directly or indirectly to the patient's diet. Likewise, longevity and happiness can similarly be attributed to the diet. Thus, the long-term effect of food will determine your health status and the appearance of your body.

- Foods can feed you or feed many. Today we live in a global community and our harvest belongs to everyone. Your diet can help support the feeding of millions or merely the feeding of the fortunate few. You can learn to eat simply so that others can simply eat.

Your garden and your shopping cart can replace your psychologist and your internist and help to solve global starvation. It begins by knowing the difference between nutrient-dense foods and calorie-

---

The Associated Press

May 3, 2006

NEW YORK -- The nation's largest beverage distributors have agreed to halt nearly all sales of sodas to public schools - a step that will remove the sugary, caloric drinks from vending machines and cafeterias around the country.

The agreement was announced Wednesday by the William J. Clinton Foundation and will also likely apply to many private and parochial schools.

"This is a bold step forward in the struggle to help 35 million young people lead healthier lives," former President Clinton said at a news conference. "This one policy can add years and years and years to the lives of a very large number of young people."

Under the agreement, the companies also have agreed to sell only water, unsweetened juice and low-fat milks to elementary and middle schools. Diet sodas would be sold only to high schools.

dense foods. You can either eat for nutrients that keep you alive at optimal levels of health or you can eat for sweetness and soothing satisfaction. When good nutrition is easy and delicious, then you will no longer dwell on the dessert menu or in the snack aisle.

Nutrients are the vital substances that create and sustain the health of your mind and body. The micronutrients (vitamins and minerals) should be densely concentrated in every meal. The opposite of nutrient-dense foods are the foods that are rich in calories and artificial flavors. These foods are commonly fast foods, fake foods and desserts. We bundle these items together as calorie-dense foods.

America has become a great proving ground for nutritional protocols. Childhood obesity, behavioral problems and diabetes are skyrocketing since the installation of soda machines and fast foods into the public schools. Our classrooms are filling with overweight children. According to the Center for Disease Control (CDC) the proportion of children ages 6–11 who were overweight basically quadrupled from 4 percent in 1971–1974 to 15.8 percent in 1999–2002.[4] Adult-onset (Type II) diabetes was historically a problem of the over 40 age group that developed blood sugar problems due to a

---

Former President Clinton and other politicians are spearheading a nation-wide change in the eating habits of our school children. Their program, The Alliance for a Healthier Generation, is a joint venture between the American Heart Association and the William J. Clinton Foundation. This alliance is working with representatives of Cadbury Schweppes, Coca-Cola, PepsiCo, and the American Beverage Association to establish new guidelines to limit portion sizes and reduce the number of calories available to children during the school day. Under these guidelines, only lower calorie and nutritious beverages will be sold to schools. (www.healthiergeneration.org)

chronically poor diet. Today children under 8 years of age are being diagnosed with adult-onset diabetes due to their fast food diets and a lack of exercise. Furthermore, the CDC reports that the proportion of adults who are obese has doubled from 15 percent in 1976-1980 to 30 percent in 1999-2002. Almost two-thirds (65 percent) of adults were either overweight or obese in 1999-2002.[5] This trend of obesity continues to rise.

Most children eat what their parents eat and both tend to eat what

---

GLYCEMIC INDEX (GI)

The glycemic index is a way of expressing how quickly a carbohydrate (sugar) is absorbed into your bloodstream. By eating foods with lower GI scores, your food will be absorbed into the bloodstream more slowly, resulting in numerous health benefits stemming from steady blood sugar levels. Eating foods lower on the glycemic index has been suggested to help lower cholesterol, prevent weight gain, lower the risk of heart disease, help manage and prevent diabetes and much more. Complex carbohydrates such as those found in whole grains, beans, fruits and vegetables are typically lower on the glycemic index. Simple carbohydrates such as those found in refined grains (white bread, donuts, etc.), processed foods, sweetened drinks or anything with added sugar tend to be higher on the glycemic index. It is best to choose foods that are near or lower than a rating of 55 on the glycemic index. Below are a few examples of data from the glycemic index. A more complete chart can be found online at: www.aliveandhealthy.com/weightlossfoods.html.

Yogurt 14	Ice cream 61
Cashews 22	Doughnut 76
Apples, raw 38	Cornflakes 81
Brown rice 55	Instant rice 90

they see on television. Our concepts of good nutrition have been either created or altered by marketing schemes of the food and restaurant industries. In this chapter, you are about to read ideas not displayed on your TV. They are simple, accurate insights about nourishment for you and your family.

You can learn to eat simply so that others can simply eat.

Adding nutrient-dense foods to your diet is as easy as walking into the produce section of your grocery store. If the food does not come in a box, needs refrigeration and has a short shelf life, then you are probably in the right neighborhood. Fresh fruits, beans and legumes, whole grains and vegetables are nutrient dense. They are great foods for the entire family.

"Fiber not Fat" is the mantra of the Happiness Diet. The fiber triad includes fruits, vegetables and whole grains. You can stay slim or become slim with huge meals of fiber rich foods, densely filled with micronutrients (vitamins and minerals). They will fill you up at every meal without unwanted weight gain. You will never feel starved when dieting on nutrient-dense foods.

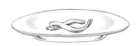 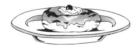

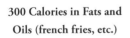

| 300 Calories in Fats and Oils (french fries, etc.) | 300 Calories in Refined Carbohydrates (donuts, candy, etc.) | 300 Calories in Fresh Fruits and Vegetables |

Fiber-rich foods receive the healthiest ratings on the glycemic index – certifying that they do not create huge upheavals in your blood sugar levels and emotions. Fiber also has the added benefit of cleansing the entire length of your intestinal tract ensuring optimal removal of waste and promoting regular bowel movements.

Oils in our diet give us that soothing, smooth creamy taste that we love. Unspoiled, healthy oils that are rich in nutrients replace the trans-fats of yesterday. Trans-fats -- found in margarines, snack foods and commercial frying oils -- increase the risk for cancer and heart disease. Ghee, olive oil and coconut oils provide optimal nutrition as cooking oils. Flaxseed oil, borage oil or evening primrose oil are consumed as dietary supplements and provide the essential fatty acids to enhance immune functions and lower the risk of chronic inflammatory diseases. All oils must be consumed in moderation, though, as even the finest oil can become problematic to your health with over-consumption.

The best time to drink your beverages is after your meal is partially digested (approximately 30 minutes after your last bite of food). Clean water, fresh juices (both fruit and vegetable) and clear teas are favorites in the Happiness Diet. Good quality milk and yogurt beverages are also important.

GLOBAL MENU PLANNING

Protein is a major fuel source for your body. It can be provided from animal sources that are expensive and, sadly, environmentally damaging. Or it can be obtained in the form of plant-based proteins that are completely friendly to the environment. In the past, scientists in America were concerned about whether vegetarians could get enough protein without eating meat. This notion has been dismissed. According to the United States Department of Agriculture (USDA), "protein needs can easily be met by eating a variety of plant-based foods."[6] It is also not necessary to combine different protein sources in the same meal. As long as your diet includes tofu, beans, tempeh, nuts or nut butters, plant-based protein can easily meet your protein requirements. The health of your body and mind favor plant-based proteins.

There are also global economic and environmental benefits to a plant-based diet. Sustaining the resources of the planet is an investment in your life and in mine. Your dietary choices can help feed others and preserve the health of the planet. Americans account for only 4 percent of the world population, but consume 23 percent of the world's beef.[7] This trend comes at a price. Using meat as a major source of food is neither an efficient nor a sustainable way to support our ever-growing global population. Processing meat uses large amounts of water, oil and gas, land and grains. These resources are conserved when diets are plant-based instead of animal-based.

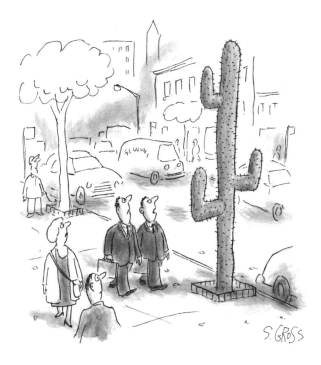

"I'm starting to get concerned about global warming."

Today, global warming is a reality. The burning of large amounts of oil in the production of meat contributes to this problem. The impact of the cattle industry on our tropical rainforests is even more significant. At a time when we need our rainforests to help reverse global warming, ranchers are cutting the rainforests down for the production of beef. More than half of the deforestation in the Amazon rainforest from 2000 to 2005 was for the purpose of livestock grazing.[8] Driving a typical American car for one day releases about 3 kilograms of gases that cause global warming. Compare this amount of gases with the 75 kilograms of gases released by deforesting and burning the Costa Rican rainforest to produce the beef needed for a single hamburger.[9] Adopting a vegetarian lifestyle is a powerful way to help end world hunger and preserve precious lands and water resources. By consuming a fresh and nutritious plant-based diet, you can help to secure a healthier, sustainable environment for this and future generations.

SUMMARY

As you study foods in this chapter, keep in mind these three key points:

A. *Foods have a powerful impact on your moods and emotions. If you keep eating the same way, you will keep feeling the same way.*

B. *Foods determine your health status, longevity and the appearance of your body. Most diseases and some deaths can be attributed directly or indirectly to the patient's diet. Likewise, longevity and happiness can be attributed to the diet.*

C. *Foods can feed you or feed many. Today we live in a global community and our harvest belongs to everyone. Your diet can support the feeding of millions or the feeding of the fortunate few. You can learn to eat simply so that others can simply eat.*

The Goddess called Happiness

The following story will give you a glimpse of possibilities that food can offer you and your loved ones. As in many great stories, it begins with a quest to find a beautiful goddess – a goddess of such purity and power that the legends have kept her secretly hidden where few would look. This goddess is called Happiness and she resides in the heart of every person. It is both a mystical secret and a profound truth — only her favorite foods and beverages will lure her out from her hiding place. Those who know this secret become established in unwavering joy.

This fully-illuminated woman is said to be the most pure and beautiful creature in all creation. She is the source of nourishment, protection and love that embraces and uplifts every seeker. Altering your diet to the foods that she enjoys will allow you to easily and consistently feel her kind, compassionate presence. If there would ever be a reason for anyone to change his or her diet, it would be in the quest of this goddess -- Happiness.

Foods Fit for a Goddess

This goddess called Happiness is a thirsty creature who loves fresh, clean water. You must quench her thirst at least five times a day, providing an offering of at least 8-10 ounces of water each time. In your transition to the Happiness Diet, begin by increasing your intake of fresh, clean water and fresh fruit juices. Herbal teas, juice without added sugar and water replace coffee, soda, and alcohol.

Joy and beauty are many times considered to be one and the same, and our goddess loves beautiful foods. Every day she desires foods containing the colors of the rainbow. Such meals may include green veggies, red veggies, yellow and orange fruits, golden ghee, earthen-colored beans, fresh roasted grains, milk, and honey.

Joy and enthusiasm are also commonly commingled. Therefore, your goddess enjoys foods that are full of freshness — the botanical equivalent of enthusiasm. In yoga, these are called high-prana (high-energy) foods. There is a saying about nutrition, "Only eat foods that will spoil or rot, and eat them before they do." If you are going to get Happiness to come out of hiding, you must offer her the freshest foods.

By no means am I suggesting a raw-foods diet; cooking your food is a useful and encouraged form of pre-digestion. An overabundance of raw foods in your diet can create a tremendous drain on your vitality in both your mind and body. Ayurvedic texts point out the importance of maintaining the fire of enthusiasm at both the metabolic and psychological levels. Mental brilliance radiates from the vital warmth of the brain. Consuming cold food or beverages can adversely shift the balance of heat from the brain to the digestive tract. When cold foods become an excessive habit in the diet, mental concentration and alertness may eventually be diminished. In the pursuit of Happiness, it is best to limit your consumption of cold foods.

In Ayurveda, foods that are easy to digest are commonly referred to as highly flammable. The radiant goddess appears in the form of the sparkle in the eyes of young lovers, the spontaneous giggles of young children, and the brilliant insights of great humanitarians. Brilliance, radiance and intensity are all metaphors for fire. To keep the glow of Happiness alive in your heart, there is no use for foods that are known to be difficult to digest. The easiest foods to digest are also the foods most recognized for promoting health and happiness. They include cooked complex carbohydrates (vegetables and whole grains), yogurt, bananas, sweet fruit (mango, papaya, peaches, deep-colored berries), cooked greens and sprouts (lentil, alfalfa, bean, radish sprouts). The most difficult foods to digest include red meat, oily fried foods, old foods (leftovers), aged cheeses (the oldest cheeses being the least favorable) and highly processed foods with chemical preservatives.) Keep your diet simple and fresh.

This goddess Happiness does not want to be overfed. Therefore, eat in reasonable quantities. End your meal feeling content rather than overly full and bloated. Start with meal portions that can be held in the palms of your hands. Weeks later these portions may shrink down.

Chew your food so thoroughly that swallowing is almost unnecessary. This will drastically decrease the amount of stress on your digestive system and greatly improve the absorption of nutrients from your meal. Thoroughly-chewed food will slide down to your stomach without a tremendous effort on your part.

> *Only eat foods that will spoil or rot, and eat them before they do.*

When it comes to healthy eating, timing is everything. The goddess Happiness wants to be fed at regular intervals. Whether your lifestyle supports four meals a day or one meal a day, do your best to eat those meals at the same time every day. Grown adults working daylight hours can fast for 12 hours every day, preferably between 7 p.m. and 7 a.m. After the evening meal, consume only clear liquids (water, juice and herbal tea) until morning. Those who wake frequently throughout the night can have boiled milk with sugar at bedtime in order to ensure a sound and restful sleep.

I have a secret for you — the goddess Happiness loves truly homemade foods. While her joy is unbounded and her love is unconditional, she is delighted by foods that you prepare yourself. Foods prepared by strangers and by machines lack the warmth and caring that only you can provide. Fresh foods easily transmit your love and compassion into the food.

The most intimate experience you can have with nature is to take a small part of it, consume it and pass it through the central core of your body. This creates a very personal bond between yourself and nature. By preparing your own food or having a loved one prepare it, you will gain more benefit from the food. Homemade food may be the biggest change of all for you. To attain and maintain happiness, have someone who loves you very much — either you or someone near and dear to you – cook and prepare your food. Gradually increase your attendance at your own dinner table. Dining in the comfort of your home will benefit you and your loved ones in countless ways. To satisfy this goddess that lies in your heart, eat simply, safely and practically. Remember, delicious, ambrosial, delectable, luscious, scrumptious food is good for everyone and pleasing to the goddess within you -- Happiness.

> A recent study in the Journal of the American
> Dietetics Association reports that children eat nearly
> twice as many calories at restaurants as they do during
> a meal at home.[10]

FOODS AND MOODS

A "happy meal" really does exist – but it is not what you think. There is no faster way to change your mood than by changing what you eat and drink. If you really want to be happy, then you cannot continue to consume foods and beverages that do not promote the very happiness you are seeking. The Happiness Diet is easy, delicious, fresh and nourishing. You will experience a noticeable difference the moment you begin to eat with happiness as the goal. This wonderful transformation to healthy meals and snacks may be the missing component in your quest for happiness.

In my medical practice, these "happiness foods" have created such a dramatic improvement in the lives of my patients that we have given it a medical term. We call it *bio-foodback*. My patients love this term because it reminds them that their mood throughout the day is simply a biofeedback indicator resulting from the food that they consume.

> *There is no faster way to change your mood than changing what you eat and drink.*

In every class I teach on self-transformation, I write on the chalkboard, "Becoming happy and healthy is not difficult, it is just different." If you want to be really happy, things are going to be a little different in every aspect. You are going to learn how to eat differently, sleep differently, breathe differently and think differently about yourself and your life. We start with food because everybody loves good food and it has a huge impact on your well-being. Later in the book, I will share with you a wide variety of methods for sleeping, breathing, meditating and contemplating – all as a means to immediately improving your life. But first, let's eat.

Food can be the cause or the cure of many illnesses. When food selection is restricted to convenience and flavor, our meals can easily become the sustainers of agitation and illness. This relationship between our food and our moods is now a well-established fact.

You *can* shape your mental states. All it takes is a little observation to notice that what you eat impacts your attitudes and emotions. Take the time to observe how your diet can potentially agitate you, make you tired and groggy, or make you calm, satisfied and mentally clear. For example, after a large serving of steak and potatoes you may feel drowsy, whereas after consuming a spicy pepper you may feel alert to the point of restlessness and irritation. If your children cannot stay calm and focused, take notice of what they are eating.

Be thoughtful and practical when selecting foods conducive to enhancing your brilliance and clarity. Treat your diet as a grand experiment and your body as the laboratory. Every time you eat something, observe the state of your body, breath and mind. The impact of food is first observed in the breathing. Foods that make your breathing long and smooth will make your mind calm and clear. Foods that make your breathing short and jerky will agitate you. Foods that make your breathing heavy and shallow produce dullness and fatigue. Soon you will feel the impact of your food on your state of mind and eventually on the state of your body.

Once you have observed all of this, ask yourself what you have learned about each particular food or meal. Was it helpful or unhelpful? If you suffer indigestion by eating a whole pizza and a quart of ice cream, don't take a digestive aid and pretend that nothing ever happened. If you disturb the laboratory of your body by consuming particular foods, remember the experience and learn from it. The next time you want a food that you know will cause problems for you, don't tell yourself that you shouldn't eat it because it is bad. Instead, ask yourself whether you want to re-live the uncomfortable consequences that you previously experienced. This way you are not placing painful rules and restrictions on your diet; rather you are making well-informed voluntary choices. The difference is dramatic. If you take the latter approach, you will find that your mind does not argue with your decision because it does not feel forced or "guilt-tripped" into the decision.

The effect of foods on your breathing, while subtle, is nearly immediate and therefore easy to observe and trace back. The effect of foods on your mind also occurs relatively quickly after eating and should still be traceable to its source. In contrast, your body is affected by the foods that you eat in ways that may take hours, several months or years to manifest. For this reason, it is useful to have some external guidance when trying to observe the effects of food on your body.

I am going to show you which foods are best for you and your family. You will see how the three main Ayurvedic constitutions require slight modifications in their meal and beverage selection in order to maintain good physical and mental health. You will not only learn what to do, but also when to do it and why. When your food and your lifestyle are aligned with the constitution of your mind and body, life will become dramatically brighter.

> *Becoming happy and healthy is not difficult, it is just different.*

MEALTIMES AND MENU PLANNING FOR HAPPINESS

Sunrise is time to *break* your overnight *fast* with breakfast. As soon as you wake, have some clean water to re-hydrate your body. Try to take time to make yourself a couple of cups of hot lemon water to help your body prepare for breakfast and your morning routine. This lemon drink consists of boiled water poured into a cup, followed by the juice of half a lemon, some honey and a pinch of salt. This hot-water-and-lemon beverage is useful twice daily to cleanse the digestive tract and stimulate a bowel movement. My patients usually need to drink two or three cups every morning and every evening in order to achieve the desired result.

Once the body is sufficiently hydrated, and after a wait of 20 minutes or more, breakfast can be consumed. An ideal morning sequence would begin with the hot lemon drink followed by stretching and a morning walk. Then comes the showering and shaving, a delicious breakfast and finally, the last-minute preparations before heading out the door to work.

For many of my patients, transitioning to a Happiness Diet means taking the time to actually *have* breakfast. Too many of us rush past the breakfast table in order to accomplish more. Nutritionally, this is like to trying to win the Indy 500 with a quarter tank of gas. We're much better off taking the time to fill the tank. I also had to be very specific in my instructions; my definition of breakfast had to be clarified in order to eliminate breakfasts consumed in the car or out of a grease-stained paper sack. Too many of my patients were eating on the run or on the drive.

A study published in the American Journal of Clinical Nutrition, April 2004, showed that consuming a breakfast high in fat (in this case an Egg McMuffin and hash browns) produces a relatively immediate and large increase in arterial inflammation. The study suggests that eating a breakfast low in fat and high in fiber and fruit may decrease your risk for heart disease.[11]

BREAKFAST

Breakfast provides foods to restart your mind and body for the new day. Cooked grains -- including oats (oatmeal), buckwheat, quinoa, and millet -- are perfect breakfast cereals. For the busy, anxious executive, millet is preferred. Millet is the only alkaline-forming grain and thus has a calming effect. Millet, vegetables, and sweet fruits will counteract the acidic qualities of a busy lifestyle by improving the alkaline level in the body.

A high quality yogurt with live culture can be blended with sweet fruits, deep-colored berries and either walnuts, cashews, or almonds for a hearty, nutritious breakfast. Granola, scrambled tofu, bran muffins, and whole grain pancakes are all useful considerations. These foods supply the protein, carbohydrates, and fats necessary to nourish your mind and body. Eggs may be used occasionally during this time of transition. (Note: recipes for breakfast can be found in the appendix.)

Mid-morning Snack

Mid-morning snacks are popular though not always necessary. Sunflower seeds, pumpkin seeds, and raisins are the best mixture for mid-morning snacking. Keep a second packet in the car for those rushed days when you need to snack on the go. For the fruit lover, apples, pears and berries should also be at hand.

Noon-time Meal

The noon-time meal is the time to have your heaviest meal of the day. When the sun is directly overhead your digestive fire is at its peak. The subtle relationship between the solar plexus in your abdomen and the sun should not be ignored. Ayurvedic wisdom encourages you to consume at this meal the six major flavors: sweet, salty, sour, pungent (spicy), bitter and astringent. This is a wonderful enhancement from the standard seasonings of sweet and salt found in the fast food diets. Gradually increase your diversity of fresh foods and flavors at lunch. The meal needs to be heavy enough to fulfill you without dulling your alertness. Thus, keep your dessert portions small and satisfying.

Bitter: any green
astringent: squash   sour: dark yogurt

Include vegetables and protein and a simple salad with a homemade dressing in your lunch. You can use eggs, dairy, beans, cottage cheese or tofu for protein. Historically, beans and grains are consumed at the noontime meal as they take longer to digest and provide you with sustenance to complete your day. For lunch, try a bean burrito or a bean and rice combination. I have included a wide variety of recipes for your lunch-time delight in the appendix.

MID-AFTERNOON SNACK

Fruits are best eaten for a mid-afternoon snack. The pectin of apples is very helpful in moving the noon-time meal further along the digestive tract. Afternoon fruits also inject a little sweetness into our busy schedules. Fresh-baked apples with cinnamon are a lovely treat to serve to your coworkers in the middle of the afternoon. This snack time could also include clear teas (herbal teas, green teas, black teas), chai and tree nut-butters, such as almond and cashew butter.*

EVENING MEAL

The evening meal is designed to help us cleanse, refresh, and relax. Warm vegetable soups, salads, baked fruits, and baked tubers (potatoes, sweet potatoes, etc.) should comprise the evening meal. Depending upon your level of activity and your constitution, you may need a much heartier meal at dinnertime. This especially applies to all people under 25 years of age because in those growing and academic years, good foods should be available as needed.

---

*Peanuts and peanut butter are discouraged because they contain aflatoxin, a neurotoxin. A recent study documented 36 different brands of peanut butter (organic included) containing aflatoxin in quantities 300 percent above the acceptable levels of safety. The effect of neurotoxins on our ability to think and on the neurotransmitters that regulate every function in our body is a well-documented concern. Therefore, tree nuts -- such as walnuts, cashews and almonds -- are the preferred choice for nut butters.[12]

AYURVEDIC MEAL PLANNING

Ayurveda provides a structured plan for choosing the foods that are best for your unique constitution. Once you identify your constitution, it is easy to design menus that are suited to your particular temperament. Foods that correspond to your constitution will supply you with the nourishment required to create psychological comfort, mental stability and the finest enhancement of physical functioning. These foods may be new to you, but keep an open mind and remember that it is imperative that your food be delicious and satisfying.

Let's begin to investigate the wonderful simplicity of Ayurvedic meal planning by briefly summarizing the unique characteristics and dietary needs of the three constitutions — the Vata, the Pitta and the Kapha.

Foods for Vata

It is no wonder that Ayurveda's first food of choice for a Vata is ghee (clarified butter). Ghee provides lubrication for all of the tissues and improves the function of the large intestine (the colon), which is known to be the physiological abode of Vata. The classic 'spaciness' of Vatas is easily resolved by helping the individual feel more grounded through the consumption of warm, soothing beverages consisting of boiled milk with spices, thick creamy soups, or protein-enriched gravies in the form of mung, toor and lentil dahl. Every main dish for the Vata constitution comes with that satisfying, grounded feeling from the addition of a small amount of ghee (1 teaspoon per main dish).

Vatas need warm food that has firmness and a light oiliness. High-quality oils, such as ghee and cold-pressed olive oil, will not make the mind dull or lethargic. This constitution is known to prefer small-sized meals and thus may need to eat four times per day. The Vatic tendency to become overly excited and scattered can be easily managed with the consumption of firm, heavy foods. Beverages should vary between fresh ginger tea and hot milk drinks, such as chai or hot chocolate. Coffee may be especially irritating to the Vatic constitution and should be avoided.

Foods for Pitta

Known for their invincible stomachs, Pittas may consume massive amounts of all foods — even impure ones, with seemingly no adverse effects. However, there are a few foods that can really enhance Pittas unwanted aspects. The classic saloon fistfight is the epitome of a Pitta being affected by alcohol. Alcoholic beverages can be particularly aggravating to Pittas, so they should be consumed in moderation, if at all. The role of the Happiness Diet for this temperament is to drive their enthusiasm and vigor closer toward joy. In time, the diehard Pittas will be comfortable limiting their intake of spicy sauces, salty chips, fat-dripping burgers and alcohol. These seemingly zesty flavors spur the Pitta into a hurried frenzy that can result in regret or error.

To cool down the fiery Pitta, begin with cooling beverages like mint, licorice, or anise teas. Anthropologists, studying desert tribes living and eating under the hot sun, found that the tribes had discovered a unique method for keeping cool — they use cooling spices in their tea and food. They can eat warm-cooked food and still have it provide relief from the heat. These secrets have allowed indigenous tribes to live comfortably in extremely warm climates without ice cubes or refrigeration. Such menus benefit the Pitta.

While Pittas can seemingly digest anything, spicy and salty foods can aggravate their mood and temperament. Sweet, refreshing fruits and lightly cooked vegetables should replace salty and spicy foods. Ghee is the best antidote for Pittic imbalances. If you are a Pitta, you can bring your metabolism back into balance by consuming small quantities of ghee with each meal.

Foods for Kapha

Kaphas would be quite satisfied living on cheesecake and ice cream, never feeling the need for a salad or hot spice. Known for their nurturing attitude, their problem-solving skills and their sweet tooth, Kaphas require an activating, energizing formulation of spices in their diet. Kaphas' tendency toward a sleepy inertia is cured with simple things like using the nasal wash (see more on this in my earlier book, *Happiness: The Real Medicine*), using black pepper with any fatty food and learning to temper their sweet tooth in exchange for mental alertness. While Kaphas crave heavy foods, they can gradually learn to eat lighter foods by increasing the spiciness in their meals.

Initially, black pepper, fresh ginger, cooked garlic, ground cumin and cinnamon are the spices used to awaken their digestive fire. Kaphas' tendency toward obesity can be prevented by discouraging over-consumption and by using spices that keep the mind alert.

Along with the aforementioned spices, it is the delicious nutrient-dense foods that are fresh and easy to digest that can further stimulate the Kapha into action. Fresh, deep-colored berries (ideally blueberries) are cleansing, delicious, and loaded with antioxidants. The dynamic life-force of fresh berries and cherries is refreshing and filling.

THE FOUR FOOD GROUPS OF MODERN TIMES

Today's modern diet seems to consist of only four food groups — fake, frozen, foreign and fast.

Fake foods are those that aren't really foods. You cannot trace them back to a specific animal or plant; instead, these foods are really chemical conglomerations made in a factory. Fake foods can include blends of meat (baloney, hot dogs, Spam) and blends of grains (chips that contain many more ingredients than just corn, wheat or potatoes). If you want sour cream and chives on your potato chips, then

I suggest you go to the refrigerator and pull out the container of sour cream and fresh chives.

Frozen foods have become a necessity for households unable to regularly shop for fresh produce. When fresh foods are not an option, quality frozen foods are preferred over commercially canned food products. The freezing process causes fewer nutrients to be lost than other chemical preservation methods. Canning heats the food inside the can, which causes a breakdown of many nutrients, especially the water-soluble vitamins.

The thawing of food with microwaves of radiation may be creating an unknown change to both the food and the person who eats that food. Historically, cooking of food has always been done by roasting, scorching or steaming the food from the outside. The radiation of the microwave heats up the cells of the food from the inside out. We still do not fully recognize the potential loss of nutrition and prana from this method. Thus, using an oven, a skillet, a grill, or a toaster is the preferred method for heating foods. Quietly and discreetly retire your microwave oven in favor of healthier cooking options.

Advanced high-tech methods of harvesting and transporting foreign foods to our local grocer provides us with many benefits but also a few concerns. During the snowy winters in Wisconsin, I can dine on fresh fruits and vegetables grown in lands much warmer than mine. Rare medicinal foods grown in other countries are now available to help you heal – an advantage unheard of 50 years ago. However, when the seasons permit, I encourage my patients to consume locally grown foods that provide the optimal level of freshness and nutrition.

Whether your foods come from your own garden or from farmers in a foreign land, there are multiple benefits to eating organically grown food. The first and most important benefit is that organic farmers are not using chemicals that harm the land, the wildlife and the water tables deep below. Clean water and a healthy environment offer you

Food Combining

Here are some food combinations to avoid for all constitutions. Certain blends of food may adversely affect your mind and emotions:

- Milk should not be consumed with sour fruit, all melons, banana, loaf breads or yogurt.
- Yogurt is not compatible with cheese, sour fruit, sourdough bread, caffeine or seafood.
- Lemon does not mix well with milk, yogurt or eggs.
- Eggs should not be combined with cheese, potatoes, yogurt or sour fruits.

greater benefits than the organic food alone. Furthermore, our ability to import foods grown all over the world has both its benefits and risks. There is a risk that imported foods could be grown under agricultural conditions that are no longer allowed in the United States. The use of herbicides, pesticides, and fertilizers, that are banned in the U.S., can strongly influence the safety of foreign foods. As consumers, it is difficult to know whether or not these chemicals were used in growing the imported foods we purchase. However, the "organic" foods will keep you safe regardless of their country of origin.

Nutritionists have multiple reservations about fast food: the quality of the food may not be in your favor, you might be traveling 30 to 70 miles per hour while you eat it, and it was probably prepared by complete strangers. Fast foods are commonly seasoned unnaturally, using excessive amounts of salt, sugar, processed grains, preservatives, fats and oils, which can lead to over-consumption.

THE IMPORTANCE OF WATER

You may notice that your thirst to drink is much more frequent than your desire to eat. This is because it is essential that your body stays well-hydrated. Since you are going to have to drink something, why not make that something clean, pure water? Not only is it wonderfully refreshing, water has a multitude of health benefits.

For example, water is essential to the lining of every internal organ and tissue in your body. Every living tissue will become sticky, obstructed, and eventually diseased if it is not well hydrated. Also, water is a carrier, providing a means for blood cells to move around the body, nutrients to move into cells and wastes to be removed. The amount of circulating water volume controls the temperature of your body and your blood pressure. Blood, lymph, and cerebrospinal fluid are all primarily composed of water.

Water uses the colon (stool), the bladder (urine), lungs (exhaled air) and the skin (sweat) as exit points for waste materials. While all four exits are equally important, modern life has diminished our opportunity to experience the positive power of perspiration. Sweating is a total body cleanse. Participating in any activity that can produce full body perspiration from head to toe will be cleansing from the inside out. This is the reason that Ayurveda emphasizes the importance of waiting to shower for 30 minutes after vigorous exercise, so that you can take full advantage of this cleansing process. It is very important to adequately replenish your fluid levels both during and immediately after your workout.

Years ago, a physician commented to me that America has ten thousand restaurants for every one colonic center. His humorous insight is sadly true. We focus the majority of our attention on taking in food and pay little attention to removing the waste matter. While I am not endorsing generic colonic therapy, my point is this: to maintain good health it is as important for waste to be safely and thoroughly removed as it is for nourishment to be received. I always advise my patients to pause for two or three glasses of warm water before retiring to the bathroom to pass a stool. An infusion of warm water makes it is much easier to pass solid matter and gas from the bowel by allowing the bowel to maintain its tone. Also, if a person uses excessive pressure to push the stool out, the presence of water prevents harm to the intestinal lining. Such a simple act — having a few glasses of warm water — can prevent diverticulitis, hemorrhoids and inflammation of the bowel.

The warmth of the water allows it to be quickly absorbed without waiting too long for the body to heat it up to the standard body temperature of 98.6 F. A cold beverage cannot be absorbed into the blood stream until the body has expended extra energy to heat that beverage to body temperature. Ayurveda discourages this avoidable waste of energy caused by ice-cold drinks.

Water is not solely important in fluid balance; it is also a form of liquid oxygen which can remove fatigue from your mind and body. Whenever you feel tired, your first response should be to drink one or two glasses of warm water. This simple elixir is both masterful and mysterious in the myriad of ways it aids us.

The body is composed of approximately 65 percent water and adults lose about three liters of water every day. The majority of this water loss tends to be replenished through food, leaving a little less than half of the fluid requirement to be directly replaced by beverages.

In order for the water to be absorbable by your body, certain trace minerals (sodium, potassium, chloride, calcium, etc.) must be present in the water. Distilled water is an example of a water source without trace minerals. When you drink water that is devoid of minerals, then your body must compensate by using its own storehouses to as-sist in the absorption of water. This results in a draining effect on the body. Drink clean water that still has all of its nutritional value.

CARBONATION, COFFEE AND COMMUNITY

The benefits of community and socializing with your loved ones are profound and should be upheld. And yet, I am the fellow who has to teach his patients to switch from a "coffee gathering" to a juice, chai or tea gathering. This new trend can be witnessed by the widespread selling of chai in nationwide chains of coffeehouses. (Chai is black tea that is mixed with boiled milk, sugar, ginger root and spices - see recipe on page 365.)

When most people think of coffee, they think of conversations, phone calls and casual morning gatherings. When I think of coffee, I think of the health problems associated with coffee, way beyond the caffeine and diuretic, stimulating effects.

In addition to being a stimulant, caffeine is broken down into uric acid, which is excreted through the kidneys. Therefore, an excess of caffeine can overtax the kidneys. However, the caffeine in coffee is of lesser concern than is the nature of the coffee bean itself. The bean consists of approximately 200 different acids, making coffee a bowel irritant. Because coffee is so acidic, it is very aggravating to the digestive system. The caffeine in coffee stimulates all of the body, including the colon, to speed up its activity. In fact, coffee enemas are touted as a method of treating constipation as it is thought that the caffeine and irritating constituents of coffee cause the bowels to increase the rate of their contractions to eliminate the irritating coffee along with all that lies in its wake.

Carbonation, most commonly associated with consumption of soda, is very aggravating to both Vata and Pitta constitutions. When any beverage is puffed full of air (carbonated), it is unsettling for Vatas. The carbon dioxide gas in carbonated beverages combines with water to form carbonic acid. Furthermore, many sodas contain phosphoric acid and citric acid (in citrus soda-pop). These slight changes in the body's pH (a measure of acidity) can cause less-than-optimal function in every part of your body.

Carbonation also has a detrimental effect on your bones. Because carbonation increases the acidity of your entire body, your body must counteract this change in pH. The best buffer for increased acidity is calcium phosphate – which is pulled out of your gut and your bones. Thus your body weakens your bone mass by using it to neutralize over-acidity from foods and excessively acidic beverages like soda pop. When you repeatedly drain your body's supply of calcium on a daily basis for years, then you may eventually lower your bone mass to the point when your bones become weak and brittle.

Soda — containing carbonation and usually caffeine — and coffee — with its irritating acidity and caffeine — are best avoided in the everyday diet. Black tea, though caffeinated, contains less caffeine than caffeinated coffee. When taken as *chai*, both the milk fat and spices, such as cardamom, act to calm the negative aspects of caffeine on your body and mind. This is a wonderful replacement for coffee. However, if you do continue your use of coffee, it would be best to add your brewed coffee to a rolling boil of sweetened milk. To the cosmopolitan, you are creating a homemade coffee latte.

The Kitchen Pharmacy

Food as a therapy is a topic that floods the bookshelves and airwaves with seasonal emphasis. For example, the warming spring rains herald the weight loss diet fads where exercising and eating less are not enough; instead, we must read 300 pages and memorize menus and charts before heading to the grocery store. The heart attack season, the dates of which are commonly determined by the media, brings television commercials and more books about how to eat right for our heart, for our blood type and for our longevity. Once again, we have much to learn and many notes to take.

As I understand it, the human race has been eating for a long time. When we eat foods that are not really foods, we commonly suffer the consequences. The ignorance of how to eat, breathe and sleep properly has caused irreparable harm to modern generations. My

Caffeine Comparison (in milligrams)
- Coca-Cola Classic (12 oz) -- 34
- Green tea (one bag in 8oz water) -- 25-40
- Black tea (one bag in 8oz water) -- 40-70
- Mountain Dew (12 oz) -- 55
- Coffee plain, brewed (8 oz) -- 135
- Starbucks' Coffee Grande (16 oz) -- 259

*Data from MayoClinic.com[13]

grandfather and many of my uncles were farmers. Options on the farm were simple and, for the most part, harmless. Their simplicity became scientific when I began my study in nutrition with Dr. Rudolph Ballentine, M.D., and Dr. John Clarke, M.D., at the Himalayan Institute in 1979. Later, Swami Rama would both simplify and embellish their teachings with broad, sweeping statements that would not be verified by medical science for 20 years or more. When reputable journals did at last publish such reassuring research, I would find myself both relieved and amazed at how much Swamiji knew.

In Rishikesh, India, in 1985, Swami Rama spoke about nutrition. He told us that various foods and spices were the gatekeepers to every metabolic function. He talked of the dangers of coffee and the benefits of turmeric and cumin. He asked us to eat with him and notice how we felt from consuming foods from his simple menu for the next several weeks. At that time, he encouraged all of us to have the experience of good food before he would expound on the scientific aspects of nutrition.

Nineteen years later, *Newsweek* magazine reported on Jan. 17th, 2005, that turmeric has the ability to "suppress genes that ratchet up inflammation." *Newsweek* referred to the benefits of turmeric in controlling the activation of the inflammation causing COX-2 gene.[14] The comments I had heard almost two decades earlier were now proven and printed. Why do we spend our time and money developing drugs that prove to be harmful, instead of trusting nature's gentle gifts, such as turmeric? At the conclusion of this chapter I have provided you with a list of spices and their benefits.

RE-STARTING THE DIGESTIVE SYSTEM

Sometimes in our life we reach a point where we have misused our intestinal fortitude to the point where we are forced to stop our daily routines of eating and snacking. This pause in consumption is necessary when your digestive system is malfunctioning and healing requires you to start over from the beginning. If this day comes, Ayurvedic wisdom will be there to greet you. You see, you were not the first one to ignore the signals of your bloating and belching as you plowed full-steam ahead into your next meal of munchies and mischief. All of us have performed outrageous nutritional escapades at home and on the road.

For the next couple of weeks your diet and your day will be different as you now re-balance and heal your entire digestive system. You will find this entire process to be easy and nourishing as you make your offerings of atonement literally into the *belly of the fire.*

Like any campfire, you are going to re-start your digestive fire as if it was a brand new fire. To clean out the fire pit, you only have to stop eating. Like your kitchen oven, your stomach is also "self-cleaning." On the eve of your first day of atonement, conclude your meal by the end of sunset and finish your waking hours with the occasional sipping of warm water that was boiled previously. When morning comes, break your fast at sunrise with the "Hot Water & Lemon Cleanse" described below. This will be your main beverage for the next three to five days. Here is the recipe:

Hot Water & Lemon Cleanse -- *To be used for 3-5 days only.*

1. Boil two quarts of water in a pot -- no microwaving. Remove from the heat. The boiling lowers the surface tension in the water, making the water easier to absorb into the body.

2. After the boiling has stopped, add the juice of two freshly squeezed lemons into the 2 quart pot of water. Boiling the lemon juice will alter and kill the enzymes in the juice. Strain the juice to prevent any lemon seeds from entering the beverage.

3. Add a small pinch of salt to the mixture, approximately 1/4 - 1/2 of a teaspoon.

4. Add approximately 1/3 to 1/2 cup of honey -- this varies according to your taste preferences. Once you know the amount that works for you, please stay with that amount. You can use real maple syrup, but honey is preferred.

5. For the Kaphic constitution, add in liquid cayenne tincture -- used in extreme moderation. About 15-30 drops for the entire 2 quarts of water.

6. Stir the elixir thoroughly and pour into a thermos.

7. Keep your lemon beverage warm and drink 8-12 ounces every 2 hours throughout your day. Always drink at least 8 ounces every 2 hours as a minimum baseline. Do not allow yourself to feel overly hungry.

8. This is *not* your only food source for the next three to five days. Also, if you are concerned about calories or carbohydrates, this might help you:

Honey has 63.8 calories per tablespoon and 17.3 grams of carbohydrates.
Maple syrup has 52.2 calories per tablespoon and 13 grams of carbohydrates.

Depending upon your personal preferences and medical history, you may find it very satisfying to use this beverage as your entire nourishment for one to three days. For the first 24 hours, this plan would be the best. Don't worry, fasting will not be your long-term lifestyle.

Like the campfire, you must feed the tiny flame very simple and easily burnable fuels. High quality yogurt that you sweeten with a fresh banana or fresh deep-colored berries is a good fuel. No grains, nuts or seeds for now. As you use the hot water and lemon beverage you will be amazed at how little food you actually need. I do believe we can all live on less food than we thought.

In regards to breaking your 24-hour fast, I would first honor whatever you normally do if you have fasted previously. If I was to offer you advice, I would start with only a few foods if possible - yogurt, fruit and warm cooked vegetables. Vegetable soups are optimal, especially when you add a teaspoon of ghee into each serving. You must do what makes sense to you. Only eat until you feel "almost" full or less. This will probably be much less than your normal habits.

Secondly, fresh crunchy vegetables are simple and satisfying - red and yellow bell peppers dipped in hummus will make an excellent snack. In the afternoon or evening, enjoy a homemade vegetable soup or stir-fry.

Ideally, use these food groups for 3-5 days. This will allow you to carefully monitor your digestion. The less food the better in the first week. (Please note that no grains are added in yet.) Over the next few days, expand your diet with tofu, broccoli & cauliflower. (No carrots yet, and still be shy on grains.) Use butter or ghee as desired. Garlic, ginger, cumin, coriander and turmeric are the best spices for cooking your vegetables and tofu.

Optimal results favor abstaining from coffee, tea, carbonation, meat and restaurant food for the next 10 – 14 days. If any food you add back into your diet causes bloating or gastric distress, please remove it again from your menu. Once your digestive fire is stronger, you can try again. Obviously, junk foods and candy are also avoided. However, you can return to eating salads at the end of the first week. Use homemade dressings if possible.

In Ayurveda, life comes from fire. The human body is said to be the kunda (fire bowl) of the Divine fire of consciousness, the spark of human goodness, the glow of the Divine from above. Accepting this metaphor for now, you can learn to view your menu as a listing of offerings that you wish to place as an oblation on the sacred fire of life that dwells within you. All that is good in life is described using metaphors of fire and light – light being the first visible sign of fire. Meals, menus and snacks all become offerings into the fire of consciousness dwelling in your solar plexus. The more precious and pure the offering, the brighter the fire of your life will glow and grow.

Your attitude is also an important part of this cleansing and rejuvenation process. You infuse your food with your emotions and attitudes while cooking and eating. The entire time you are cooking, eating and digesting, the food is listening. Have a blend of delightful conversations, enchanting music and family fun at each and every meal. The optimal musical tunes are those sung by all before or after the meal. My father always kept his baritone ukulele leaning in the corner of our dining room – at any moment throughout dinner he could break into song.

Day 1	Hot Lemon Drink Snacks* (optional)
Day 2	Hot Lemon Drink Snacks (optional) Cream of vegetable soup (optional)
Day 3	Hot Lemon Drink Snacks (optional) Cream of vegetable soup (optional)
Day 4	Hot Lemon Drink Lunch - Vegetable stir-fry, Tiger sauce (optional) Snacks (suggested)
Day 5	Hot Lemon Drink Lunch - Vegetable stir-fry, Tiger sauce (optional) Snacks (suggested)
Day 6	Breakfast - Yogurt and fresh fruit (blueberries, strawberries, bananas) Lunch - Tofu, vegetable and cashew stir-fry Dinner - Cream of vegetable soup
Day 7	Breakfast - Yogurt and fresh fruit Lunch - Mung bean soup, whole wheat toast (optional) Dinner - Cream of vegetable soup, whole wheat toast (optional)
Day 8	Breakfast - Yogurt and fresh fruit Lunch - Scrambled tofu, whole wheat toast (optional) Dinner - Toor dal, brown rice (optional)

Continued on next page

Day 9	Breakfast - Yogurt and fresh fruit
	Lunch - Lentil soup, whole wheat toast
	(optional)
	Dinner - Tofu, vegetable and cashew stir-fry,
	brown rice (optional)
Day 10	Breakfast - Yogurt and fresh fruit
	Lunch - Toor dal with mango, whole wheat toast
	(optional)
	Dinner - Coconut vegetables, brown rice
	(optional)

*Snacks can include apples (fresh or baked with cinnamon), bananas, cherries, grapes, fresh red or yellow bell peppers dipped in hummus, and fresh nuts.

(cashews, almonds or walnuts).

Recipes for all meals listed here can be found in Appendix C.

CONCLUSION

Feeding the goddess called Happiness . . . .

Like every good friend and every great parent, the goddess Happiness lovingly accepts every gift you offer. I believe her presence in our lives and at our dinner tables is needed now more than ever. Knowing your sincerity in your search for a healthier, happier life, I offer you menus that can help you heal the past and the present, as you bravely stride into the future you create. You will find the menus in the appendix.

As you watch those around you glow with the fire of joy from good food and good friends, I hope this chapter has inspired you to see your meals, menus and snacks in a new light. Delicious, delectable, scrumptious living. Live it.

CHAPTER SUMMARY

A few basic principles on how and what you eat will guide you toward the quality of life you seek.

- *Foods have a powerful impact on your moods and emotions. If you keep eating the same way, you will keep feeling the same way.*

- *Foods determine your health status, longevity and the appearance of your body. Most diseases and deaths can be attributed to the patient's diet. Likewise, longevity and happiness can be attributed to the diet.*

- *Foods can feed you or feed many. Today we live in a global community and our harvest belongs to everyone. Your diet can support the feeding of millions or the feeding of the fortunate few.*

To live a healthier lifestyle, follow these simple dietary ideas.

- *Reduce and consider removing fast food, junk food and overly-processed foods from your diet. Home-cooked meals will make it easy for you to avoid foods with added salt or sugar, refined sugars and refined grains.*

- *Limit dairy and meat consumption (especially ice cream and aged cheese).*

- *Add fruits and vegetables.*

- *Add whole grains.*

- *Switch to healthy oils.*

- *Replace soda, alcohol, coffee and sweetened juices with water.*

- *Enjoy your meal in a calm peaceful environment. Take time to chew your food thoroughly. Try to eat at regular times throughout the week.*

Strengthening your Digestive Fire

There are three simple things you can do before and after every meal to improve your digestion. The entire process of digestion is based on reducing your foods to tiny molecules that can enter your blood stream and nourish your body. Once your food particles are thoroughly chewed and reduced in size, then they flow through the entire length of your intestines. Making the absorption of these nutrients easier and increasing the ease with which the remaining foods and waste are removed from the body is called "increasing your digestive fire."

- Before and after each meal do three simple things:

  1. Bend - From a standing position bend over and touch your toes or ankles three times.

  2. Twist - From a standing position hold your feet steady as you twist your torso to look behind you -- three times to the left and three times to the right. Then repeat the toe touches.

  3. Breathe - Take your seat at the table and breathe slowly sixteen times, expanding your abdomen with every inhalation. As you exhale, pull your abdomen toward your spine. This breathing practice increases the pressure in your abdominal cavity to encourage the absorption and removal of matter in your digestive system. Then take a few sips of water and begin your meal.

- CHEW YOUR FOOD THOROUGHLY.

- ENJOY YOUR MEAL IN A FRIENDLY AND RELAXED ATMOSPHERE.

- FIFTEEN MINUTES AFTER YOUR MEAL IS COMPLETE, REPEAT THE STRETCHING EXERCISES AND THE BREATHING EXERCISE.
  1. Bend - From a standing position bend over and touch your toes or ankles three times.
  2. Twist - From a standing position hold your feet steady as you twist your torso to look behind you -- three times to the left and three times to the right. Then repeat the toe touches.
  3. Breathe – Sit down and breathe slowly sixteen times, expanding your abdomen with every inhalation. As you exhale, pull your abdomen toward your spine. Then take a few sips of water.

These simple exercises will improve your digestion and elimination of food. Chew the food, move the food, absorb the food, and eliminate the unabsorbed remainder.

*notice how your breathing changes after eating certain foods
* food contains energy - so making positive feelings b/4 + while making meal

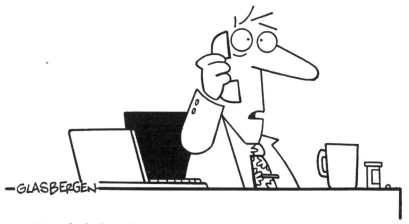

"My job is giving me migraines, high blood pressure, chest pains, and bleeding ulcers. I'd quit, but I like their health plan."

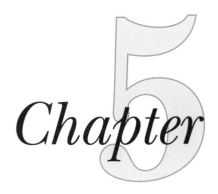

Chapter

Hatha Yoga
Fitness for the Body, Breath and Mind

B ring up the subject of exercise and you're bound to get a lively reaction out of most people. Some people love their morning run, while others dread anything that may require them to leave their couch. Regardless of where you fall on this spectrum, exercise is an essential ingredient in a happy life. Life is movement. Just as water that sits still becomes stagnant, our body and mind can easily slip into the stagnation of discomfort, depression and disease if we do not stretch and exercise sufficiently.

WHY EXERCISE?

Research has finally affirmed what every good doctor has observed for centuries. Happy people are healthy people. Happy hearts are healthy hearts. Observing indicators of physical health – such as blood pressure, heart rate, cortisol (a hormone released in response to stress) levels, immune system function, as well as occurrence of chronic diseases -- with respect to mental health, has left researchers with one clear fact: *your psychological well-being and your physiological well-being are inextricably linked.*

Depression has been closely linked to heart disease. The concept of the "broken heart" is more real than you may have imagined. Doctors are beginning to understand that not only do their patients need to get healthy, they also need to get *happy.* Exercise has the ability to help you reach both of these goals.

You may need to encourage and even discipline yourself in order to gather the momentum to start and maintain an exercise program. Just knowing the well-established benefits of regular exercise should be encouragement enough. These benefits include increased cardiovascular health and decreased risk of heart disease, increased strength and flexibility in your joints and muscles, increased strength in your bones, lower blood sugar levels, improved function of the immune system, maintenance of a healthy weight, decreased risk of many chronic diseases such as breast cancer, colon cancer and diabetes, increased life expectancy and decreased likeliness of depression and anxiety. The bottom line? Exercise will improve your overall health, state of mind and quality of life.

> *Exercise will improve your overall health, state of mind and quality of life.*

Exercise is particularly useful in cultivating a happy mind. From a biochemical point of view it is easy to understand why. Exercise activates and balances the levels of neurotransmitters (serotonin and norepinephrine) associated with depression and general reactions to daily events. Also, in a phenomenon commonly known as "runner's high," exercise stimulates production of neurotransmitters (endorphins) that result in feelings of well-being.

Through the wisdom of yoga science, additional benefits of exercise are unveiled. Memories, emotions and any physical or mental stresses or traumas are all stored, not only in the mind, but also in the tissues of the body. When we exercise and stretch properly, we allow the body to process, resolve and release these impressions. This fact is easily illustrated by observing your state of mind while stretching. Notice how feelings of discomfort or irritability, that may have been present at first, are resolved as physical tension is removed. Furthermore, while exercise improves the physical circulation in our body, yoga exercise improves the *pranic* (energetic) flow of our body.

How to exercise

What is proper exercise? How much should I exercise? These are questions whose answers are less agreed upon by modern research.

In 1996 the U.S. surgeon general recommended a minimum of 30 minutes of physical activity most days of the week to reduce the risk of many chronic diseases. In 2002, the Institute of Medicine (IOM) recommended at least 60 minutes a day of "moderately intense physical activity" for adults. Other recommendations range in between. Finding the time to exercise can be difficult in today's hectic world. Ironically, the days when exercise seems impossible are the days when it may be precisely what you need. Even a five-minute walk or a quick neck roll and forward bend can be helpful and can relieve a tremendous amount of stress. The most important thing to remember about exercise is that any amount is better than none.

> *The most important thing to remember about exercise is that any amount is better than none.*

Similarly, almost any type of exercise is better than none. However, different types of exercise will yield different results. It is important to consider what results you are seeking before you choose an exercise routine.

In America, much of the fitness industry has been influenced by the world of "body building" – which focuses on appearance, not performance. When you want to show clear definition of a specific muscle, then you exercise that muscle or group of muscles in isolation in order to gain maximum engorgement of the muscle. This is not fitness, but purely for show. In everyday life, when we perform practical actions such as walking, lifting, running, pushing and jumping, we do not use our muscle groups in isolation. Rather, our whole body works in synchronicity to provide balance, strength and grace to our movements.

Jon Hinds, a renowned fitness instructor, has been studying, teaching and writing about fitness for more than 20 years. When he pointed out the absurdity of exercising my muscle groups in isolation, and the fun of moving my entire body, my interest in fitness finally returned. For 25 years I had been a desk-ridden homeopath and teacher, although previously I was an active martial artist for many years. The exercise

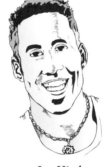

Jon Hinds

schemes sold on the television – I bought several – were just not much fun to do alone in my living room. Jon introduced me to a mentality toward fitness training that is enjoyable and makes sense.

He warned me that even if I avoided the "ab-rollers" and the weight lifting machines of the world, I may still fall prey to the "core stabilization" programs and become fixated on core stabilization. "There are whole programs on core training," Jon said to me. "I don't agree that you should solely focus on strengthening the central core of your body. To do so is good, but it is not enough. In my mind your core is your whole body. Instead of saying core, I use the term *alignment stabilization*. Whatever is the first point of resistance in your exercise, be it your feet or hands or head, from that point on, you have to be stabilized."

Jon went on to explain why. "If I am in a handstand, my hands are the first point of resistance – resisting the ground and the force of gravity. My hands and feet have to stabilize first and foremost when pushing a car. If they are in poor alignment, the next joint up the line will be in poor alignment too. For example, people with flat feet have ankles that are in poor alignment - they lack stability. It is impossible to have stable knees if your ankles are out of alignment - it's a domino effect - your ankles, your knees and then your hips. In reality, if you have back pain, you might have a foot problem. If you exercise with misalignment and don't correct it, your problems will come to the surface quicker in the form of pain and possible disability. You could work your core all the time, but if you aren't working it correctly, from the extremities in, then you are missing the boat. It's impossible for the domino effect not to occur."

I asked Jon how he works to prevent this domino effect. "One of the things I do is I intermix yoga with modern fitness styles," he replied. "I teach you to stabilize the entire body, beginning with your first point of contact with resistance – which is usually the ground or floor. The greater stability you have at each joint the less likelihood you have of injury. Yoga has been around for thousands of years and focuses on alignment of the whole. The better we place our head, feet, hand and butt on the ground with more stability and more squareness to the ground, the more prepared we are for a dynamic natural exercise, such as running, jumping and climbing.

"When you start to do hatha yoga, you naturally learn how to stabilize your joints. Adults lack this basic stability today and then when they try to do some basic calisthenics they are terrible at them.

Consequently, they are more apt to get injured. Much of the fitness industry furthers this problem by not acknowledging the fact that you should stabilize on your own. Instead, they provide you with machines to sit on."

Jon went on to point out that even in the practice of yoga it is important to be mindful of how you do your practice, and explained how an instructor or partner can be useful in this respect.

"A good yoga instructor provides you with essential feedback. You can go through a yoga sequence, but if you are not aware that you are out of alignment, you will adapt to mal-alignment and you will continue to do the movement sub-optimally. For those who do not have access to live instruction, if you do your exercises with regularity and awareness, there is a good chance that because you are constantly repeating each movement in a systematic fashion, eventually you will self-correct in the end. However, if you get feedback on certain areas that are collapsing and you strengthen those weakened muscles, then over a shorter period of time you will perform more efficiently.

"Optimal feedback means working with an instructor or partner. A mirror does not provide enough feedback and mirrors can promote the 'appearance' mentality of body building. I want you to focus on fitness-based function and performance, not appearance.

"The feedback you can get from a partner should come in the form of encouraging internal resistance. To start with, your partner can put their hands on different parts of your body that are collapsing so that you can work into those areas and strengthen them. Eventually you will develop an internal awareness of your body. Bring your attention to your areas of weakness so that you can work into them. Pain is an amazing feedback mechanism. If your lower back is painful, try to resist into it, push into it, because these are the muscles that have collapsed. You want to engage into them instead of hanging in that position. Don't hang! Instead straighten, extend and expand!

Lengthen and expand that area. Engage your muscles from the inside out, learn how they feel. Your tone, strength and function will improve over time as you activate, contract or expand your body. Remember, engagement usually begins in the hands and the feet. But more importantly, please remember that freedom of movement is the ultimate goal.

"Everyone has imbalances in the body. Often times it is created through habit. All I do is try to create more balance in the body through basic movement and internal awareness. Yoga is the perfect exercise for working the synergy of the whole body."

Jon continues to introduce yoga and fitness through his seminars and classes throughout the nation. He gave life to my hatha practice and continues to encourage me to push back from my desk everyday and go move, stretch and expand.

Thus, in this chapter we will introduce and enthusiastically recommend a unique and comprehensive system of exercise that has withstood the test of 5,000 years. This system is referred to as *hatha yoga*.

HATHA YOGA — FITNESS FOR THE BODY, BREATH AND MIND

In hatha yoga there is a systematic series of postures and stretches that help strengthen and rebalance the body. What makes this system unique is its underlying philosophy. In yoga, all methodologies are aimed in the direction of self-transformation and self-understanding. The human body can be a wonderful tool or a cumbersome burden. It can be a source of joy or a source of misery. To transform it into a vessel for happiness, you will have to understand how both joy and misery are created. At first glance, this may seem obvious. You know that you won't be very happy when your back is in spasm or your neck is so stiff that it is giving you a headache. But there are subtler indications of a happy or unhappy body that come long before crippling back pain. One indication of imbalance is a change seen in the breathing pattern. All of us know that we are breathing and thinking beings. But in truth, most of the time you are not consciously breathing, rather your breath flow is automated in accordance to your most consistent style of breathing. When your physiology changes during sickness or stress, the harmony of the breath is disrupted and muscle spasms and tightness can be the result. Unaware of this importance of breath regularity, we miss the warning signs that an altered breath pattern is trying to announce.

A happy body is one that is not just free of pain, but one that also maintains a healthy, open and relaxed posture. Your posture should lift your ribcage slightly, relieving excess pressure from the lungs and heart. This allows for deep diaphragmatic breathing and healthy functioning of the heart. Hatha yoga is a systematic series of stretching, balancing and strengthening *asanas* (postures) and exercises that allows you to achieve this kind of body.

There are three main components to physical fitness: 1) energetic and physical strength, 2) cardiovascular endurance and 3) flexibility. Hatha yoga addresses all three. The word hatha refers to a blend or balance of the sun and the moon, or the active and passive energies of the body. Therefore, it makes sense that practicing hatha should leave the body balanced and address your needs for stretching, strengthening and aerobic activity. However, hatha alone is not recommended as a sole source of aerobic exercise. I encourage everyone to spend at least 30 minutes every day walking, jogging, swimming or biking as a regular component of your exercise routine.

To develop a loving relationship with your hatha practice, it may be helpful to think of it as your own personal massage therapist. Just as a massage therapist would, the asanas of hatha release muscle spasms.

In these newly-relaxed muscles, circulation increases and the tissues of the body rejuvenate as blood brings in fresh oxygen and nutrients and carries away waste products. Muscles that are in spasm can pull your body out of its natural alignment, distorting your posture by hiking up a shoulder or a hip. Hatha fine tunes the body by releasing these distortions and restores a proud and comfortable posture.

Twisting, bending, stretching and holding your body in the unique asanas of hatha gives your body a massage that even the most skilled therapist couldn't provide for you. That's because hatha massages and rejuvenates all of your internal organs. It heats and lubricates deep inside achy stiff joints to restore your range of motion. A good hatha routine is like getting a massage from the inside out.

While it is true that exercise will help you in achieving happiness, exercise alone is not enough. True and lasting happiness can't be attained simply by running a six-minute mile or becoming so flexible you can put your toe in your ear. The sages who gave us the gift of hatha yoga understood this. Although it is a valuable set of exercises on its own, the real potential of hatha is revealed when it is applied as a foundation for practicing the subtler exercises in the greater discipline of yoga science. These subtler exercises are *pranayama* (breathing exercises) and meditation. When these three practices - hatha, pranayama, and meditation - are combined properly, the flower of happiness will most certainly blossom in your heart.

A good hatha teacher is one who has studied all of the aspects of yoga and understands where hatha fits into this broader picture. Such a teacher may spend just as much time providing you direction for your breath and the focus of your mind as they do providing direction for your physical body. Our body has amazing potential for recovery and healing if it is allowed the opportunity. Proper use of the mind and the breath provide the environment for this potential to come forward.

Jamming to your favorite tunes on your iPod or Discman may make exercise seem like more fun, but providing the silence necessary for your mind to turn its focus inward is infinitely more rewarding. As you turn your attention inward you will begin to feel the natural rhythms of your body. You will feel which muscles need attention. You will notice your breath and be able to begin to use it as a tool.

At all times during the practice of hatha be aware of your breath. Short, shallow, jerky breaths stimulate the sympathetic nervous system and promote tension in your body. Smooth, deep, diaphragmatic breathing stimulates the parasympathetic nervous system and allows your body to relax. The complete practice of hatha always includes breath awareness and pranayama. These ancient exercises have a profound ability to balance, cleanse and rejuvenate the physical and energetic body. In addition, during every stretch, it is helpful to bring your awareness and your breath to the area of your body being stretched. Obviously the physical gases of your breath are restricted to your lungs and airways. However, if you imagine your whole body being capable of breathing and filling with air, you will find that the energetic or pranic qualities of the breath reach far beyond the lungs and can be brought to any area of the body. When this kind of attention is given to any area of your body, pain and fatigue are washed away in the tide of your breath.

After practicing hatha in the manner just described, you'll find that your body becomes a delightful home, your mind is turned inward and quiet, and your breath is calm and serene. Every practice of hatha ends with a relaxation exercise to fully assimilate the benefits of the workout.

This all may sound wonderful enough as is, but the full experience of hatha does not stop here. The comfortable body, quiet mind and serene breath gained through hatha and pranayama were intended to be the foundations on which one can build a stable mind and sturdy senses through the practice of meditation. It is on the path of meditation that you will find the true treasure of yoga. When your body, breath and mind no longer distract you, then you will find this treasure. You will find yourself. You will find happiness.

MENDING THE BODY

The most basic definition of the term "yoga" is "union." Creating a union between your body, breath and mind has countless benefits both psychologically and from the viewpoint of productivity and efficiency.

I am going to provide you with a full hatha routine to get you started. Keep in mind that even if you don't have time for this whole routine, something is always better than nothing. Even sitting at your desk is no excuse for not stretching. Without even requiring you to get up, a neck roll, a side bend with your arm overhead, and a gentle spinal twist are perfect stress-busters for your back, neck and shoulders. You can increase your abdominal pressure by simply bending forward with your back straight so that your abdomen lies on your thighs, breathing deeply as you hold a seated forward bend. If you work on a computer, your wrists and forearms will rejoice from simple wrist circles. Gently guide your wrists through their full circular range of motion and feel the blood begin to flow again as those tense, typing muscles let go. Providing some self-massage to the forearms will give you added relief.

Let's start with simple warm-up exercises that will unite your breath and your body. As you learn to move and bend with your breath, you will be so pleased with how your mind starts to settle down and take direction from you. Keep in mind that hatha is not a competitive sport. Turn your attention inward. Remain aware of your breath. Relax and breathe serenely in every posture. Most research indicates that the stretch receptors of muscle tissue take about 30 seconds to respond to a stretch; thus hold your stretch until your stretch receptors respond. Your hatha practice is the most comprehensive way to know and heal yourself.

THE WARM-UP ROUTINE

Stand up. Breathe through your nose. This routine starts with a "half-neck roll." While exhaling, drop your chin to your chest, keeping your shoulders back. Bring your awareness to the center of your forehead.

As you inhale, slowly sweep your chin up toward your left shoulder; during exhalation, sweep your chin back down to the center of your chest.

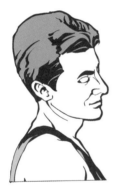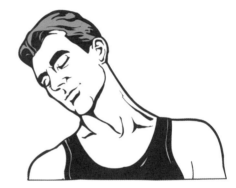

The half-neck roll

On your next inhale, swing your chin toward your right shoulder; during exhalation, swing your chin back to the center of your chest. Continue this neck roll, repeating it three times in each direction. Keep your awareness in the center of your forehead. The final movement of this exercise involves lifting your chin back up and off of your chest while inhaling, allowing your head and neck to return to the upright position.

Next come shoulder rolls. Roll your shoulders in circles, three times in both directions — forward and backward. Allow your breath to flow smoothly and evenly through your nose. Keep your awareness in the center of your forehead.

Now repeat the half-neck roll three times in each direction. Continue to keep your awareness in the center of your forehead.

Begin horizontal arm swings. From a simple standing posture, inhale as your bring both of your arms up to shoulder level with your palms facing downward. Swing your arms in front of you and behind you 12 times, keeping them horizontal to the floor. Each time you swing your arms, alternate which arm is on top. As you become more limber, your palms may touch each other behind your back. Keep your awareness in the center of your forehead.

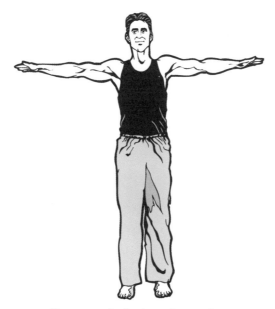

The posture for horizontal arm swings

Now repeat the half-neck roll three times in each direction. Keep your awareness in the center of your forehead.

And now for the grand moment - the forward bend. This simple stretch is known to address all of the issues of fear, addiction, and survival. Start in a simple standing posture. Let the weight of your head pull you to the floor in this movement. Begin by exhaling your chin to your chest. On your next exhalation, slowly bend toward the floor, keeping your chin on your chest and your awareness in the center of your forehead. Take a few deep breaths as you bend. It is fine to bend your knees in the beginning if you are feeling too much of a stretch. Cross your forearms and hands with each other and hang for a while. You will feel the stretch throughout your arms, legs and spine.

When you are ready to return to a standing position, slowly rise up starting with your toes, ankles, calves, and thighs. Unfold your arms allowing them to hang to the floor, and keep rising upward. Straighten your knees. Inhale as you are standing up. Keep your chin on your chest. Once you are standing erect, on your next inhalation, raise your chin off your chest and stand tall.

Repeat the forward bend three times. When you are hanging over, keep your breath flowing gently through your nose, keep your chin on your chest, and your awareness in the center of your forehead. Hold the position for 3-10 breaths and then gradually rise back up to standing position.

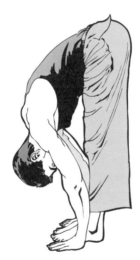

The standing forward bend

Now, repeat the half-neck roll three times in each direction. Keep your awareness in the center of your forehead.

Begin overhead side stretches. Using one arm at a time, inhale as you raise your arm from your side up to shoulder level, with your palm facing the floor. At shoulder level, rotate your palm toward the sky. As you continue to inhale, move your arm straight overhead until your arm is next to your ear. On your next inhalation, stretch your arm upward, and then while exhaling, side bend at your waist to the opposite side. Hold the stretch for three breaths and then lower your arm to your side as you exhale. Repeat the stretch for a total of three times with both arms. Keep your awareness in the center of your forehead.

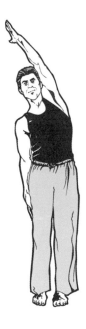

A standing side-bend

If you only have 10 or 20 minutes, stop at this point and go on with your day. Just this simple routine is enough to quiet your mind, leaving you relaxed and focused. Free from the chains of pain, stress and fatigue, you will find yourself more productive and full of joy. If you have more time, continue on with the solar salutation and a brief series of revitalizing asanas.

The Solar Salutation and Other Revitalizing Asanas

The solar salutation is a flowing set of asanas that awakens your solar plexus – the core of your digestive power and endurance. It addresses every major muscle group, leaving you relaxed, refreshed and energized. The solar salutation is the traditional beginning of a hatha practice. You can perform this sequence in a slow, smooth and graceful manner – bending, bowing and rising up once again to newfound feelings of flexibility and freedom. Repetitions of the solar salutation can also be done quickly, jumping from one posture to the next, heating the body and providing cardiovascular exercise. Luke Ketterhagen, a certified yoga instructor, will share with you his expertise in hatha to guide you through the solar salutation and the following asanas.

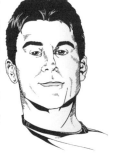

Luke Ketterhagen

The Sun Salutation

Mountain pose: Stand tall with your feet hip-width apart and your arms at your side.

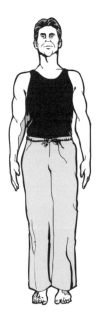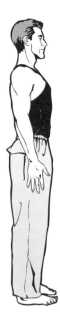

Prayer position: Bring your hands up to your chest so that your palms press together in front of your heart.

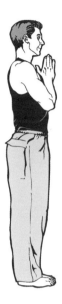

Overhead stretch: Inhale and raise your arms over your head stretching tall toward the ceiling as you press your feet into the ground. This is a full body stretch.

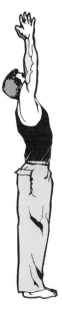

Standing forward bend: Spread your arms out to your side and exhale as you fold forward from your hip joints. If your hamstrings are very tight, a slight bend in your knees will help release your lower back. Take a few breaths and allow your upper body to release closer to your legs.

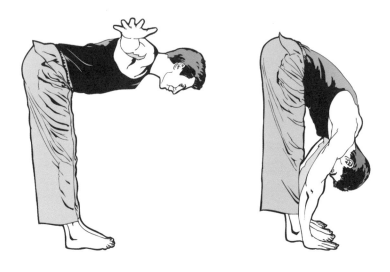

Right leg lunge pose: Inhale and step your left leg back leaving your right leg forward, between your hands.

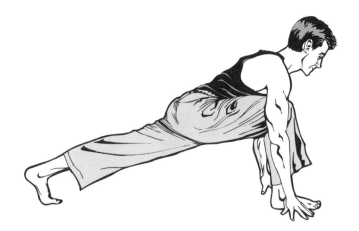

Downward facing dog pose: Exhale and step both feet back to this inverted "v" pose. Press your hands and feet down evenly. Lift your hips and then lower your heels to stretch the backs of your legs. Lastly, relax your neck and the area between your shoulders.

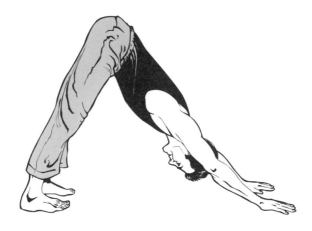

Plank pose: Inhale and lower your hips down so that your body comes in to a high push-up position.

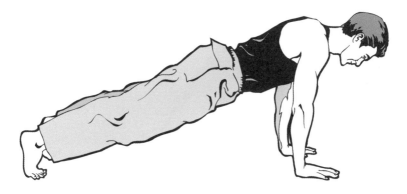

Cobra pose: Exhale and slowly lower your whole body down to the floor. Inhale and press the front of your pelvis and the tops of your feet into the floor while using your lower back muscles to lift your chest off of the floor. (Do your best to avoid the natural urge to use your arms here – this posture helps build your lower back strength.)

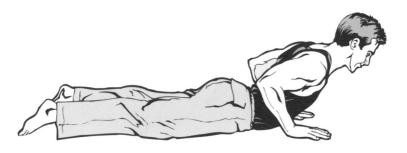

Downward facing dog: Exhale, press your hands down to lift your body back up into the downward dog position again.

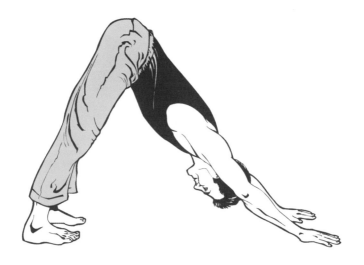

Left leg lunge pose: Inhale and lunge your left leg forward, placing it between your hands.

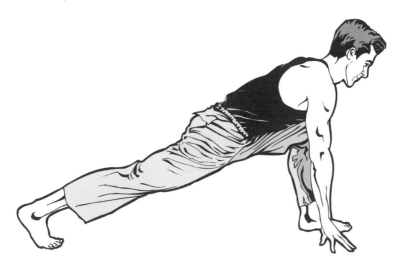

Forward bend: Exhale and step your right foot forward to meet your left. Relax your upper body toward your knees as you come into a standing forward bend again.

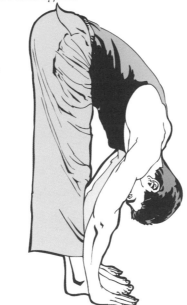

Overhead stretch: Inhale and lift up to standing with your arms stretching toward the ceiling. Stretch your whole body.

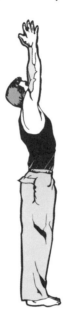

Prayer pose: Bring your hands back down and press them together in front of your heart.

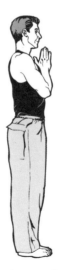

Salute the sun and watch your internal sun awaken!

Warrior One: The warrior is a posture of strength and victory. Breathe and feel the flow of power and vitality that is generated in this posture. Warrior One is wonderful to re-awaken your personal power and self-esteem.

Stand tall with your legs hip-distance apart. Step your right foot back about 3-4 feet. Turn your right foot out slightly. Lunge your left knee forward as you move your right hip forward. Extend your arms up, but keep your shoulders dropped down away from your ears. Your gaze is forward, steady and relaxed. Breathe deeply 8 – 10 times and feel your body releasing down through your hips and stretching up through your arms and torso. Switch sides and stay in the final pose for as many breaths as you did on the first side.

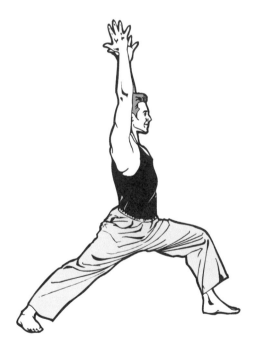

Abdominal Squeeze: This exercise is unparalleled in its ability to awaken your solar plexus, improve digestion, stoke your metabolic fire and massage all of your visceral organs.

To begin, stand with your feet hip width apart. Place your hands on your legs, just above your knees. Transfer the full weight of your upper body through your arms and onto the support of your legs. As you exhale, pull your abdomen in toward your spine creating a concavity in your abdominal area. This should feel like you are squeezing the internal organs of your abdomen. On inhalation, relax your abdomen, breathing deeply into your belly. Continue to squeeze on exhalation and relax on inhalation. After a few breaths, begin to slow your breath down and deepen your contraction as you exhale and your expansion as you inhale. Repeat this 10 to 20 times.

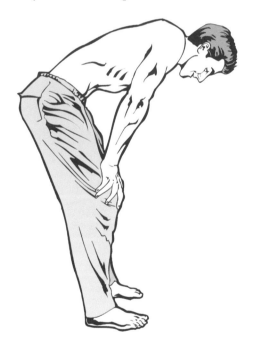

Butterfly: Sit on the floor with the soles of your feet together in front of you and your heels drawn in close to your pelvis. Clasp your hands around your feet and press your knees down toward the floor. Lift your lower back to straighten your spine and bring your weight evenly to your bottom. Breathe deeply and continue to feel the resistance of your hips and inner thighs release.

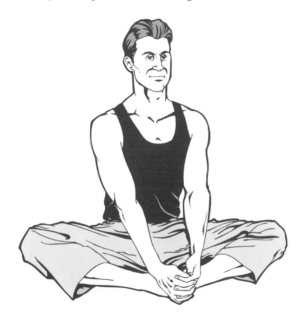

Cat and Cow: Get onto all fours. Your wrists are directly under your shoulders and your knees directly under your hips. As you exhale, push your hands down and lift your back up. Tuck your tailbone down, drop your chin toward your chest and pull your abdomen in toward your spine. As you inhale, arch your back downwards. Lift your chest so that you are looking up. Press your sit bones up toward the ceiling behind you and feel your abdominal area drop and expand toward the floor.

Repeat this exercise several times, lengthening your breath and maintaining the coordination between your movements and your breath. Arch down on your inhale and round up on your exhale.

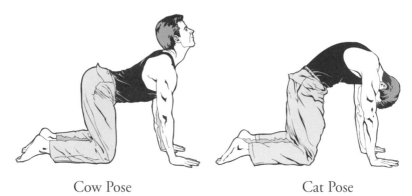

Cow Pose   Cat Pose

If you wish, you can add leg movements to these postures. In coordination with your exhalation and the rounding of your back (cat pose), bring your right knee in toward your nose. This will strengthen your abdomen and stretch your lower back. In coordination with your inhalation and the arch down of your back (cow pose), extend your right leg back and lift it off the floor until it is straight. This will strengthen the back of your leg, buttocks and lower back. Repeat 8-10 times and then switch sides for the same amount of reps.

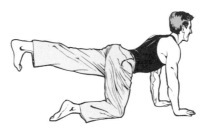

Cow Pose with Leg Extension

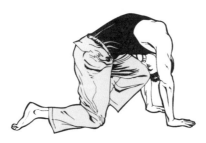

Cat Pose with Knee to Forehead

Child's pose: Begin on all fours and then sit back on your heels. The tops of your feet are flat on the floor underneath you. Allow your upper body to relax down toward your thighs. Relax your neck, bringing your forehead toward the floor in front of your knees. Stretch your arms out in front and rest them on the floor. Your abdomen presses against your thighs as it expands with each inhalation. With each exhalation allow your body to settle closer to your legs. Stay here for up to 1 minute as your low back releases.

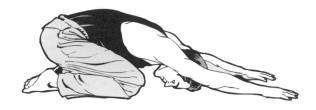

Bridge pose: Lie on your back with your knees bent and your feet 4-6 inches apart. Rest your arms by your sides, palms down. On inhalation, press your feet into the floor and slowly lift your hips off of the floor. Continue to slowly raise the rest of your spine off the floor one vertebra at a time in a rolling motion. Press your palms and forearms into the ground, as shown. Bring the weight of your upper body onto your shoulders by gently rocking from side to side. Hold this posture and breathe deeply into your abdomen. Stay here for up to 1 minute and then stretch out on the floor to rest your back.

(In this pose, your neck can feel crunched if your shoulders are too close to your ears and your chin is tucked into your throat. To release your neck, bring your shoulders down away from your ears and slightly lift your chin.)

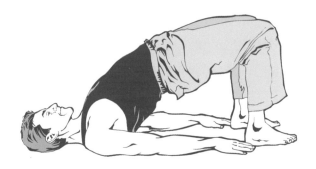

Reclining leg cradle: Lie on your back with your knees bent and your feet hip-width apart. Cross your right ankle over your left thigh. Reach your right hand through the space created by your legs. Clasp your hands together interlacing your fingers so that you can hold onto the back of your left thigh. If your hands don't come together, use a sock, towel or strap to hold the back of your thigh. Draw your left thigh toward you as far as is comfortable for you. Relax your back and shoulders down and allow your head to return to the floor. (Note: If there is a deep arch in your neck you may prefer to use a small cushion under your head to lengthen the back of your neck). Breathe deeply and watch your right leg and hip release. As your right side opens, you may be able to gently pull your left leg closer to your body. Stay here for 1 minute, and then switch sides and repeat for the same amount of time.

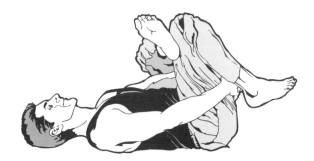

Reclining twist: Lie on your back and hug your knees toward your chest. Leaving your legs in this position, stretch your arms out to your side and rest them on the floor with your palms facing down. Bring your knees to your left and rest your legs on the floor – your left leg settles to the floor and your right leg relaxes on top of your left. Turn your head to your right. As you hold this posture, relax your upper body and watch your right shoulder blade relax back toward the ground. On an inhalation, come back to center and then repeat the stretch on the opposite side for the same amount of time.

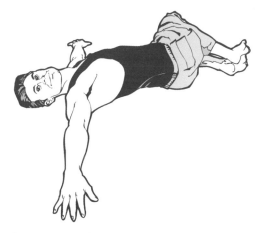

Systematic relaxation in the corpse pose: Lie on your back with a small cushion under the back of your head. Rest your arms flat on the floor with your palms facing up. They should be slightly removed from your body so that they don't actually touch your sides. Separate your feet so that they are a little more than hip-width apart, allowing your pelvis to fully relax. Close your eyes and feel your body sink into the floor.

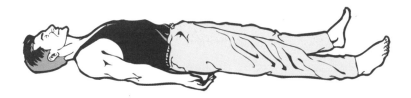

Now survey your body and see if your body is still sending any signals to your brain. If so, it means that there is still discomfort somewhere. Make the minor adjustments necessary to fully rest. As the breath deepens, watch your body accept the support that the floor provides. When the body is fully supported by the floor, you will feel complete stillness. Now let your breath become your major focus. Breathe slowly and smoothly through your nose and mentally follow the rise and fall of your abdomen.

Once you are comfortably resting in the corpse pose, it is time to begin a systematic relaxation. If you have the time, the 61-point relaxation exercise that is outlined in chapter 7 is an excellent way to end this routine. If you want something shorter, use the following alternative.

A Brief Relaxation Exercise

Bring your awareness to the crown of your head. On your next exhalation, breathe as though your breath is flowing from the crown of your head, down through your body and out the soles of your feet. On your next inhalation breathe as though your breath is flowing in through the soles of your feet and up through your body to the crown of your head. Repeat this for a total of three breaths. After the third and final inhalation, exhale down from the crown of your head again, only this time, stop at your ankles. Then, inhale up from your ankles to the crown of your head again. Breathe from the crown of your head down to your ankles and back up to the crown of your head for a total of three times. In the same manner, always beginning on an exhalation, breathe from the crown of your head down to your knees and back up to the crown of your head. Then, breathe three times from the crown of your head down to your perineum at the bottom of your pelvis and back up to the crown of your head. Breathe three times from the crown of your head down to your belly button and back up to the crown of your head. Breathe three times from the crown of your head down to the center of your chest and back up to the crown of your head. Breathe three times from the crown of your head down to the center of your throat and back up to the crown of your head. Breathe three times from the crown of your head down to the center of your eyebrows and back up to the crown of your head.

Upon completion of this relaxation exercise, please take a moment to observe the state of your body, breath and mind. Before you return to your daily activities, lie still for a few more breaths. Then start to awaken your body by gently wiggling your fingers and toes. With your eyes remaining gently closed, rub your palms together to create some heat between them, and then cup your warm palms over your eyes. Open your eyes into the warmth of your palms and slowly remove your hands when you are ready. Then bend and lift your knees and gently roll over onto your left side to rest there for a few minutes before slowly pushing yourself into a seated position. Once you are in a seated position, stand up and resume your day.

Chapter Summary

- *In everyday life, when we perform practical actions such as walking, lifting, running, pushing and jumping, we do not use our muscle groups in isolation.*

- *Whatever is the first point of resistance in your exercise, be it your feet or hands or head, from that point on, you have to be stabilized.*

- *The greater stability you have at each joint the less likelihood you have of injury.*

- *Engage your muscles from the inside out; learn how they feel. Your tone, strength and function will improve over time as you activate, contract or expand your body. Remember, engagement usually begins in the hands and the feet. But more importantly, please remember that freedom of movement is the ultimate goal.*

- *In hatha yoga there is a systematic series of postures and stretches that help strengthen and rebalance the body.*

- *The complete practice of hatha always includes breath awareness and pranayama. These ancient exercises have a profound ability to balance, cleanse, and rejuvenate the physical and energetic body.*

- *Turn your attention inward. Stay aware of your breath. Relax and breathe serenely in every posture. Your hatha practice is the most comprehensive way to explore and heal yourself.*

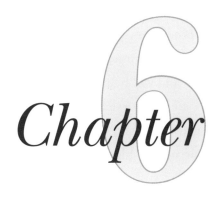

Chapter

Homeopathy: The Energy Medicine

W hen lifestyle changes and determination are unable to free you from major blockades to happiness, then homeopathic medicines may be the answer.

Modern medicine has finally documented how your long-term habits alter your metabolism. These metabolic changes continue until one day your metabolism actually supports and maintains the problems that you are trying to overcome. It is not uncommon in the lives of my patients to do all the right things – dietary changes, relaxation exercises, vitamin and mineral therapy, and physical exercise – and still find their metabolism continues to create their unwanted emotions. When this common scenario reaches my office door, homeopathy can be the godsend that my patients have been seeking.

For more than 200 years, people worldwide have been using homeopathic medicines to regain a healthy metabolism and healthy emotions. When the body's metabolic momentum needs to be corrected, I have found that homeopathic medicine is the most powerful, fast-acting, and completely safe therapy in the world.

Everyone has some issue that seems impossible to overcome. For some it may be a physical malady -- like migraines or arthritis – and for others it may be a mental health issue -- like anxiety or insomnia. This book is intended to introduce you to solutions for these concerns and will help you find freedom and happiness. In this chapter you are going to learn specific homeopathic remedies to release deepseated habits and emotions that may have held you captive for years or decades. This is the miracle of homeopathy.

WHAT IS HOMEOPATHY?

Homeopathy is a word that was coined by a German physician named Samuel Hahnemann (1755 – 1843) in the 1790s. The word homeopathy is a combination of two Latin words: *homeo* -- meaning the same or similar -- and *pathos* -- meaning tragedy or suffering. Thus, homeopathy literally means *similar suffering.* This word was the best way Hahnemann could describe this new medical methodology that he had discovered.

> *Homeopathy often helps people overcome physical and psychological problems when other therapies have failed and the problem seems impossible to overcome.*

The amazing discovery of homeopathy began when Hahnemann was working as a medical translator and physician. In 1790, Hahnemann was given the task of translating Cullen's *Materia Medica*, which included the most current medical therapies. (The term "materia medica" literally means the materials of medicine. William Cullen was a Scottish physician and author.) During his translation project, Hahnemann stumbled upon a very astringent Peruvian bark called "cinchona" or "china" that was commonly used in the treatment of malaria. Cullen's book noted that this bark contained quinine and concluded that "china" was helpful for malaria due to its astringent (drying) properties. In his translations of this work, Hahnemann made a bold footnote that he did not believe the bitterness or astringency of the Peruvian bark made it helpful in treating malaria. Instead, he believed that there was something unique and special about the bark.

Then Hahnemann did something very unusual – he used his body as a laboratory. In an effort to further understand this Peruvian bark, he decided to consume it. He ground the bark into a powder and diluted it with sugar. He repeatedly consumed the bark dilution until finally he developed symptoms. Hahnemann's amazing discovery was that his symptoms from too much Peruvian bark were very similar to the symptoms of malaria. However, he did not have malaria. Once he stopped taking the bark he became well again. This experience of repeatedly consuming a substance until symptoms develop is called a "proving."

Hahnemann took his findings a step further. He also discovered that very diluted extracts of Peruvian bark, when given to patients ill with symptoms similar to his own experience, completely cured their illnesses. This astonishing finding inspired Hahnemann to experiment with other herbs and minerals.

He started "proving clubs" with his medical colleagues and their families in order to understand the nature of various plants and elements. During his lifetime, he alone verified the unique nature of 90 different natural substances. This experiential knowledge of how the raw plant or herb affected human beings was organized into a text he called his "Homeopathic Materia Medica." Just as with the Peruvian bark, he matched the illness and experience of his patients with his personal Materia Medica, which described how people responded to various substances. Once he found a good match, he gave the patient a very diluted dose of the natural substance and the patient had a curative response.

How Remedies Are Made: Serial Dilutions

Natural Substance   1 Drop

1 Drop

1 Drop

1 Drop

1X

2X

3X

4X

Mother Tincture

9 Drops
Pure Alcohol

9 Drops
Pure Alcohol

9 Drops
Pure Alcohol

9 Drops
Pure Alcohol

More Potent, More Dilute

Each vial is shaken vigorously after each dilution is made.

Homeopathic Dilution

To understand the safety of homeopathy, you need to understand the method of homeopathic dilutions. It is a science that is not fully understood by today's modern scientists, but can be verified by over two hundred years of clinical case studies.

When you dilute a substance, you first have to start with the substance itself. Let's take a plant such as pulsatilla, the wood flower. First, the pharmacist grinds the plant, macerating it in alcohol, which produces an herbal tincture, also known as the "mother tincture" of pulsatilla. From this mother tincture, the pharmacist then begins a series of serial dilutions.

The first dilution begins with an empty vial in which nine drops of water (or alcohol) are added with just one drop of the mother tincture. Thus, the first vial -- which we'll call Vial 1 - has a total of ten drops (nine drops of water and one drop of the original substance).

The pharmacist then shakes this dilution vigorously a minimum of 16 times. The shaking between each dilution is what makes the homeopathic remedy active. This process of shaking is called succussion. It must be done between each dilution in order for a homeo-pathic remedy to be made. If the succussion is not done between each solution, the dilute solution will have no medicinal power.

Next the pharmacist takes *one drop* from Vial 1, and adds it to a new vial (Vial 2), with nine drops of pure water and succusses it 16 times. This is called a 2x dilution of pulsatilla.

Then the pharmacist takes one drop out of Vial 2 and adds it to Vial 3, then adds nine drops of pure water and succusses it. Vial 3 would then be labeled as a 3x homeopathic dilution.

If the pharmacist continues these serial dilutions 23 times, always adding one drop to nine plain drops of water, this yields a 23x dilution. The 23rd dilution is significant because according to the 18th century physicist Amadoe Avogadro, zero molecules of the original substance will be contained in the 23rd dilution. Therefore, at a 23x dilution, *zero molecules of the original mother tincture exist in the vial!*

With such a minute, non-physical dose only the energetic essence of the original tincture remains. Such a highly diluted medicine offers you freedom from side effects and toxicity. This amazing benefit is not available in any other system of medicine. A homeopathic remedy that clearly matches the symptoms of the patient will stimulate the body's healing forces to awaken, rise up and rebalance the mind and body, thus curing the ills of the patient. If there is not enough similarity between the remedy and the patient's symptoms, then the homeopathic remedy may have little to no effect on improving the patient's condition.

Homeopathic remedies go even further than 23x in their diluting process — all the way up to 100,000 dilutions. The incredible finding of Hahnemann and the homeopaths who followed him was that the more dilute the tincture, the more powerful its effect. This fact has made the modern understanding of homeopathy even more perplexing for today's scientists. Modern science cannot detect a single molecule of the original mother tincture in the 30x dilution vial, nor can it explain how more dilute remedies have a stronger, more curative effect on the patient.

Furthermore, there are centesimal dilutions in homeopathy. These homeopathic remedies, denoted with the letter "c" (for centesimal), are made from dilutions of 99 drops of pure water instead of 9 drops, resulting in a vial having 100 drops in total. Both the decimal and centesimal dilutions of homeopathic remedies have more than 200 years of clinical experience as well as many modern clinical trials proving that homeopathy is not a placebo medicine. This evolutionary understanding requires modern science and quantum physics to enjoin into a higher refinement of medicine and healing. Most commonly, homeopathic remedies are prescribed at the dilutions of 6c, 9c, 15c, 30c, 200c and 1000c.

MATERIA MEDICA

The 90 substances tested in Hahnemann's lifetime can now be found in the Homeopathic Materia Medica, along with additional medicines tested by Hahnemann's students and present-day homeopaths. The total number of remedies is now more than 2,000. The Materia Medica is a thorough listing of every homeopathic remedy and the symptoms they are known to heal. The Homeopathic Materia Medica has also been very insightful in understanding modern diseases.

For instance, many Americans consume coffee on a daily basis. The Materia Medica listing for coffee shows many mental symptoms. The listing for coffee cruda, the unroasted coffee bean, has the symptom of sensitivity to all sensory stimulation. Under the mental symptoms, the Materia Medica lists irritability, gaiety, excitement, impressionability, being filled with ideas, quick to act, and tossing about in anguish. It also lists symptoms affecting the head, such as a tight pain anguish. It also lists symptoms affecting the head, such as a tight pain made worse from noise and smell and sensations as if the brain were torn to pieces from a nail driven into the head. If you have ever seen people go through coffee withdrawal, and they get headaches, you may see that they have head pain similar to what is described. Coffee is also known to cause toothaches, which are temporarily relieved by holding ice water in the mouth. Coffee can cause symptoms that include hasty eating and drinking, excessive hunger, intolerance of tight clothing and sleeplessness on account of mental activity.

So, if my patient was a small child who was teething, felt better chewing on chips of ice and had too much mental excitability to be able to stay asleep at night, I could say that this child's symptoms are most similar to the symptoms of too much coffee. This little child has not consumed any coffee at all, but the child has symptoms similar to the suffering of coffee intoxication. Applying Hahnemann's theory of letting likes be cured by likes, I would prescribe coffee in a homeopathic potency as the remedy most likely to give the child relief from teething.

Homeopathic Remedies for Grief and Sadness

Homeopathic medicines have the unique ability to help you get through difficult situations with style and grace. Sometimes, when you get stuck in a bout of sadness and grief, homeopathy can help release pent-up feelings that you have suppressed and bring you back to a state of happiness.

Ignatia

I remember going to my first funeral - maybe everyone does. I definitely remember the lump in my throat. I was 11 years old and I was choked up with sadness and grief. My dad said that the lump happens to everyone.

A couple decades later I looked into this phenomenon, which is called *globus hystericus* — basically the hysterical sensation of a lump in the throat. It is a sensation that all of us have felt at one time or another. Later I would learn that the "lump" is a key symptom for determining certain remedies for grief.

When I first started studying homeopathy with Dr. Dennis Chernin, M.D., in Ann Arbor, Mich., one of the first patients that I observed in his clinic was suffering from the long-term effects of unresolved grief. The hour-long interview was cut short by 50 minutes. Dr. Chernin immediately wrote a prescription for homeopathic Ignatia 200c before the fellow could complete his story. With the patient still present, Dr. Chernin turned to me, "Ignatia (St. Ignatius' Bean — Ignatia amara) is the most famous remedy for grief in homeopathy. It addresses the elements of hysteria and spasms - like a lump in the throat - brought about by grief. This fellow, like many others, could have benefited from taking Ignatia years ago when tragedy struck his family. During times of overwhelming grief and loss, which everyone in the entire human race experiences, Ignatia is fantastic."

> *The miracle of Ignatia is in its ability to help patients release deep-seated grief.*

Dr. Chernin went on to explain that Ignatia is especially useful for people who are overly emotional and sensitive. The miracle of Ignatia is in its ability to help patients release deep-seated grief that has been difficult or impossible for them to resolve on their own. Instead of processing the grief and loss, the momentum of these emotions become trapped inside, causing sensations of spasm and cramping. The patient's colitis began immediately after a tragic car accident and increased after his wife's funeral. Five years later the cramping still hadn't stopped and it brought him to Dr. Chernin's door. Dr. Chernin was confident that Ignatia would resolve this spastic quality and psychologically help his patient regain his spirit to live and enjoy life.

A few weeks later, the patient returned looking more energetic and happy. His colitis was completely cured and his emotional outlook was much brighter. I was astounded by this amazing result, which Dr. Chernin had prescribed after only 10 minutes.

Years later I have now seen so many miraculous cases where deep grief and sadness were resolved using Ignatia. When my patients complained of this same "lump in the throat" that I had experienced as a child, I knew Ignatia would be the perfect remedy for them and would bring them closure and relief.

Because grief and loss are such universal experiences, I want to share with you a little more information so that you can help yourself, your family or a friend overcome long-lasting sadness quickly and easily using this homeopathic remedy.

Key Symptoms Remedied by Ignatia:

- Any ailment (illness or problem) that began from the experience of grief, sorrow, bad news, homesickness, disappointed love, shame, or embarrassment
- Hysteria with hysterical symptoms, such as numbness, tingling or acute paralysis
- Refusal to be consoled
- A desire to be left alone to weep in seclusion
- A strong desire to avoid crying due to the person's underlying fear that if he starts to cry, he will not be able to stop
- Deep sobbing

- Desire to travel and move around
- A sense of relief when walking in the rain
- Headaches from grief
- Lump in the throat (globus hystericus)
- Heavy sighing and yawning
- Insomnia or excessive sleepiness from grief

Ignatia is commonly sold in health food stores at a potency of 30c. My patients commonly take a 30c dose twice a day until they feel that their grief or sadness is under control.

NATRUM MURIATICUM

Ninety percent of the time, when the classic symptoms of grief and hysteria are present, Ignatia will be the miracle cure. However, there are those people who express their grief by becoming silent and withdrawn, with no signs of hysteria. In these cases, Natrum muriaticum (Natrum-mur) will be the likely cure.

> *Natrum-mur can be a wonderful solution for those who suffer deep grief and hide within themselves.*

A few years back, a 15-year-old girl named Sandy was brought to my office. Her boyfriend had committed suicide and in the past month since his death her grief had driven her deeper inside. She spoke clearly and articulately about her misery, "I felt it should have been me who died because I was depressed, not him. I feel so depressed that I do not want to get out of bed. What is the point of life? You will just die anyway." She stopped and stared off into the distance.

Tears were starting to form and her mother was becoming restless in the chair beside her. Sandy's tear-stained eyes turned back in my direction. "Why even get close to people? Either you get hurt, or they get hurt. And people are going to die and go away."

She became silent. I waited.

Finally her mother broke the silence. "She is not responding to anything the school counselors told us to do. She is getting weak, and she's lost more than 30 pounds. She dwells on his death."

"Is she doing anything unusual? Craving anything peculiar?" I asked, searching for clues to the right remedy.

"What's really odd is that she's craving salt. Of my three kids, she was the girl with the sweet tooth. And now all she likes is salty chips and pretzels."

It would have been impossible for Sandy and her mother to realize, but they were describing the exact symptoms that can be treated by homeopathic Natrum-mur. This homeopathic remedy, made from table salt, covers the ailments from grief and disappointed love when expressed as silence, depression and complete withdrawal. This individual dwells on past grief and humiliations in a manner that makes her hesitant to have further contact with society. Such a person is very sensitive to noise and music and seeks to isolate themselves where no one can offer them a consoling hug. They must do everything possible to avoid being humiliated or embarrassed. The grief may last for an abnormally prolonged amount of time. Natrum-mur also addresses the issues of social awkwardness commonly seen in adolescents who lack the comfort and social skills to communicate with their peers. The young person, unable to comprehend or adjust to sudden loss, may completely shut down as an initial reaction to grief and loss. Commonly, a person needing Natrum-mur may start to bite their fingernails or develop headaches or even migraines as a reaction to stress and grief.

I gave my patient, Sandy, Natrum-mur at a 1M potency (M=1,000 dilutions) and had her return a few weeks later. Two weeks later her smile was proof enough that Natrum-mur had worked. Her mother demanded her to give testimony immediately as they sat down.

"I could tell the difference right away," she reported. "There are no more ups and downs. The roller-coaster is over. She is on a much more even keel. She still has some down days, but they are normal compared to her past experiences. Her concentration is better and she takes a greater interest in her high school and athletic goals."

Sandy beamed as her mother reported the changes. "And my concentration at school is a lot better," she chimed in. Once again, Natrum-mur had worked its magic.

Key Symptoms Remedied by Natrum Muriaticum:

- Silent grief
- A tendency to be closed and withdrawn
- Depression with the potential for suicidal feelings
- A desire to be overly proper but often without the social skills required
- Very loyal and sympathetic to others
- A refusal to divulge secrets — the keeper of confidences
- Easily wounded or offended by insults and criticism
- Unable to stop dwelling on past grief and humiliations
- Strong desire to always be on time and always be perfect
- Adverse to consolation — feels too embarrassed to accept a consoling hug during times of grief and sadness when such embracing would be socially appropriate
- Bites fingernails, frequent hangnails
- Feels aggravated from long periods of time in the direct sun
- Known for being a serious person; a child who behaves "like a little adult"
- Headaches or migraines that are worse from light, sun, or from reading

- Easily cracked lips
- Sensation of a lump in the throat
- A craving for salt
- Inability to urinate in public restrooms unless completely alone
- Insomnia caused by thoughts of grief and disagreeable things

Natrum-mur can be a wonderful solution for those who suffer deep grief and hide within themselves. The result is usually a dramatic shift outward and a cheerier disposition. When someone who is suffering from grief becomes stuck inside themselves, Natrum-mur can save them from their despair. Commonly, health food stores carry homeopathic Natrum-mur at 30c potency. For deep-seated grief a potency of 200c or 1M may be needed once a week. These higher potencies are usually only obtained from a homeopathic pharmacy.

SEPIA

One of my first patients that I saw privately, while training with Dr. Chernin in 1982, was an overwhelmed housewife. She rapidly shifted her attitude from sarcastic, cutting remarks about the status of her family and the world to sitting perfectly still, sullen and lifeless. Arguments and confrontations brought her to life, as she unleashed her vicious tongue. As one of my very first patients, she was not making me, the new homeopath, very comfortable at all. Through her bitterness I could still glimpse her sincere outreach, looking for a hand up, as if she wanted me to pull her out of the rut that encased her life.

Her chief complaint that brought her to my door was her self-proclaimed alcoholism of over 15 years. But my immediate focus was on her shifting states of mind going from lifeless to enraged in less than a second.

Sepia officionalis is the remedy for deep-seated inertia and the collapse of soft tissue strength. When life events have brought an individual's world to a standstill, it may be the solution. Sepia is the ink juice of the cuttlefish used by the fish to hide from a predator, offering a brief opportunity for escape.

When people are frightened and overwhelmed, and their response is to become completely still, it is called the "possum response" to stress. They feel dead inside and like a corpse, they do not move. They may report the feeling of a black cloud or sense of darkness surrounding them. They are frightened and do not know in which direction to go with their life. They commonly feel guilty and isolated from their loved ones, feelings that may appear in the form of detachment and indifference toward their family and friends. They become weepy, irritable, and sarcastic. They feel better when completely alone and when they engage in vigorous exercise or activity.

My patient clearly had all the signs of a Sepia case. I sent her home with Sepia 200c, hoping my next visit with her would be more pleasant. A month later she returned and was doing much better. She no longer had these rapid shifting moods and was better able to cope with opposition. Her alcohol consumption had stopped because her desire for the beverages had completely disappeared. Sobriety came easily.

Over the years, Sepia has been one of the most common remedies in my remedy kit. Many people respond to stress by "playing possum," holding still and playing dead. This response often results in low self-esteem and deep-seated fears about the world. In these cases, Sepia can help to bring them out of their shell and back to a state of wellness.

Key Symptoms Remedied by Sepia:

- Isolation and withdrawal
- Weakness
- Laxness in the tissues, causing sagging, prolapse, constipation and sluggishness
- Indifference and disconnectedness
- Mental dullness
- Weeping without knowing why
- A tendency to be easily angered and irritable
- An aversion to company
- The tendency to feel better when left alone
- The tendency to feel better from vigorous exercise and activities
- A sensation of emptiness in the stomach that is not improved by eating
- Aversion to being touched
- Urine leaks from coughing, laughing or sneezing
- Cold hands and feet
- Hormonal imbalances caused by stress and inactivity
- A bearing down sensation, as if the entire womb was going to prolapse, during the menstrual cycle

Sepia is a common remedy that can be found in health food stores at a 30c potency. For more extreme cases, the 200c potency is usually found at homeopathic pharmacies.

REMEDIES FOR COLLAPSE, EXHAUSTION AND FATIGUE

One of the greatest privileges in medicine is being able to release an individual who has been imprisoned for years by a syndrome or situation that seemed incurable. In the realm of fatigue and exhaustion, a well-selected homeopathic remedy can breathe life and vigor back into a person who has been bedridden from overwhelming fatigue. Any homeopathic remedy that matches that patient's symptoms can bring about a curative response. Over the years, I have seen five different remedies that most frequently match the various phases of collapse and fatigue. Three of these remedies are known as the "acids of collapse" and the other two are classically known for relieving fatigue and symptoms of the flu.

PHOSPHORIC ACID

Karl came to my office the week before his final exams at the end of his first year of college. His mother described him as an enthusiastic lad who wanted to be an engineer like his father. He threw himself into his studies with relentless energy. His first semester went very well, but come spring, he had faced major challenges in mathematics.

While we talked, Karl sat in his chair, emotionless. He was completely indifferent to his mother's comments and my gentle, probing questions about his health. He had burned himself out trying to be a top-grade student. His mother told me that he had now lost interest in everything except for listening to music. His fatigue began approximately six weeks earlier when he did poorly on his midterms. He had also developed diarrhea in response to the stress at school.

Seeing this state of collapse, his mother brought him to me, looking for a miracle. His final exams were days away and Karl had no desire to study. He would constantly remind himself of his potential failure. His state of indifference, hopelessness, and fatigue were the classic symptoms of needing the homeopathic remedy of Phosphoric acid. This college freshman had started his academic year with vigor and high hopes and now sat before me quiet, withdrawn, and disappointed. He was grieving as if his whole world had died because of his poor midterm grades.

I gave Karl one dose of Phosphoric acid 200c and the very next day his mother reported that the "old Karl" was back! He became more alert, more hopeful, and more focused.

> *The state of indifference, hopelessness and fatigue are the classic symptoms resolved by Phosphoric acid.*

Karl relapsed into his withdrawn fatigue in the middle of summer, but one more dose of the remedy brought a lasting cure.

The typical Phosphoric acid patient is fatigued and drained to the point of appearing lifeless or indifferent. While this is also a remedy for grief, it is more strongly indicated for a total collapse that may be caused by a debilitating illness, such as diarrhea or mononucleosis; more than just grief alone. Patients appear to be apathetic, dull, and depressed. They are forgetful and slow to answer any questions. They appear to be non-reactive to the world around them and are commonly fixated on music or television, yet oblivious to everything else.

Key Symptoms Remedied by Phosphoric Acid:

- Severe fatigue
- Indifference
- Hair loss or change in hair color (from grief)
- A tendency to weep easily
- Loss of vital bodily fluids
- Weakness from sexual excess
- Painless diarrhea

Please remember that Phosphoric acid, as a homeopathic remedy, is completely devoid of any of the original acid molecules. Therefore, this remedy is completely safe at a 200c potency that would commonly be found in a homeopathic pharmacy.

MURIATICUM ACIDUM

I would probably never have had the chance to meet Max if it weren't for his hemorrhoids. In medicine, I guess that is not such an unusual introduction, but for Max, hemorrhoids were the least of his problems. He was a 62-year-old business executive known for his constant struggle to make his business succeed. Downsizing and the reality of competitors using more affordable overseas work forces had presented Max with the challenge of his life. Several months earlier the financial reports on his company warned him that his business would most likely go under.

Shortly after that, Max rapidly declined into a bedridden state. The chief financial officer of the company was a friend of mine and had tried, on several occasions to get Max to see me. It was only when Max's hemorrhoids became so painful and he felt too weak to go through another rectal surgery that Max's wife finally brought

> *The collapse that occurs in patients needing Muriatic acid is seen as a profound physical weakness.*

him to my office. He was one of the few people I had seen who had to be brought in a wheelchair. Max was in a state of total collapse. Even in the wheelchair, he would slide down as if trying to slip to the floor and go back to sleep. This wonderful executive felt hopeless and dead.

I had treated many pregnant women for their large, bluish-purple, grapelike hemorrhoids with low doses of Muriatic acid. I knew how well it worked. So upon completing my examination of Max, during which I found the same classic hemorrhoids, I immediately prescribed Muriatic acid 200c. Both the condition of his body and his state of total collapse demanded it.

Within 10 days his extremely painful engorged hemorrhoids were gone, and his fatigue was lifting. At the end of six weeks he had accepted his company's fate, resumed his role as CEO and began to dismantle his firm. This single dose of Muriatic acid cured his fatigue and his hemorrhoids with no other treatment given.

The collapse that occurs in patients needing Muriatic acid is seen as a profound physical weakness. The patient may be unable to rise up in the bed to greet family members. He may sleep more than 18 hours of the day. Homeopathic literature classically describes this patient as one who is so weak that when you prop him upright in a bed or in a chair, he slowly slides back down to a horizontal repose. This muscular debility can be a comprehensive problem that affects the entire body or may appear in the form of localized areas of paralysis or weakness. Muriatic acid is also a classic remedy for hemorrhoids that are swollen, tense, dark blue and extremely painful to the slightest touch.

Key Symptoms Remedied by Muriaticum Acidum:

- Paralysis or severe weakness
- Hemorrhoids that are swollen, tense, dark blue or purple and painful
- Sadness
- Irritability
- A state of collapse, as seen in septic conditions
- Excessive sleepiness

Keep Muriatic acid in mind any time you see people who have lost their energy to the point of complete paralysis. This remedy, often given at 200c, can be a lifesaver.

PICRICUM ACIDUM

Picric acid concludes our triad of the "acids of collapse." This is the remedy for complete collapse of the intellect. The old homeopathic books refer to this state as "brain-fag," and today we call it complete burnout. In this state, the mind loses its ability to read and concentrate. Practically all patients who need this remedy are overpowering intellectuals, students, writers, and researchers. Quite simply, they have stretched their problem-solving capacity to its limits.

The kind of collapse treated by Picric acid is commonly caused by mental exertion from over-studying and experiencing overwhelming intellectual strain. The mind becomes dull, tired and unable to concentrate any further. The patient cannot remember what he read within minutes after reading.

> *Picricum acidum is chiefly for those highly intellectual people who have gone way beyond their capacity.*

Often, he also has physical weakness made worse from any kind of exertion or even from passing a stool. Rest, sleep and Picric acid in homeopathic potency will greatly improve the patient's condition.

Key Symptoms Remedied by Picricum Acidum:

- Collapse from mental exertion
- Dull mind
- Tiredness
- Inability to concentrate
- Difficulty reading
- Weakness from physical or mental exertion

Picricum acidum is chiefly for those highly intellectual people who have gone way beyond their capacity. Usually higher potencies are needed to revive their mental brilliance. This remedy is not commonly found in health food stores and is usually obtained from a homeopathic pharmacy.

KALI PHOSPHORICUM

A sense of nervous dread was his modus operandi. Single and in his mid-40s, Roger lived in a world of worry and weakness. He was oversensitive to every event and encounter. Roger was so nervous and so easily startled that the slightest touch would result in a massive jump, causing everyone around him to startle. I think his friends and family described him as a high-strung worrier. No matter what was going on in his life, he felt like he was unable to cope with the situation. This would consistently lead him to a state of collapse, very often resulting in a call to my office.

Roger had been through a smorgasbord of therapists over the past 20 years before my supervising physician referred him to me. He was chilly, restless, and nervous. Any unexpected noise or touch, no matter how benign, startled him in such a violent manner that made me think his life was at risk. His chronic fatigue, chronic anxiety and headaches demanded the homeopathic remedy Kali-phosphoricum.

Due to his intermittent use of anxiety medications, Roger's homeopathic remedy had to be repeated frequently throughout the year, but it always brought him good results in the form of improved self-esteem, a decrease in his overly exuberant startling, and a full return to feeling vigorous and dutiful. Any course of therapy is easier to select and prescribe when no other medication is being used. Today this ideal situation is rare.

I start my patients on a remedy and have them continue all medications and therapies. Once I see improvement exceeding their past experiences with other treatments, then we might consider the gradual elimination of other medications. It is important to understand that this change in medications requires the care and skillful monitoring from the entire team of physicians and family members.

The remedy Kali phosphoricum is for mental fatigue. Patients' oversensitivity to noise, suspiciousness and nervousness is caused by fright, sleeplessness, fear, or grief. They are chilly and feel greatly depleted. Their headaches are caused by, and made worse from, mental exertion. They are tearful, wanting to avoid conversation and feel that everything is too overwhelming for them.

> *The essence of Kali phosphoricum patients is the "jumpy" nature of their nerves and the mental exhaustion brought by fatigue.*

Key Symptoms Remedied by Kali Phosphoricum:
- Oversensitivity to noise
- Suspiciousness and nervousness
- Sleeplessness
- Chilliness
- Headaches
- Tearfulness
- Avoidance of conversation

The essence of Kali phosphoricum patients is the "jumpy" nature of their nerves and the mental exhaustion brought by fatigue. A quick trip to the local health food store for Kali phosphoricum 30c will quickly resolve their jumpiness and fatigue.

GELSEMIUM

In the world of homeopathy, Gelsemium is the classic remedy for the flu. If your symptoms are a match for the specifics of Gelsemium, you will delight in the rapid freedom you gain from these seasonal ailments by taking this wonderful remedy.

Gelsemium is useful for weakness and drowsiness brought on by sudden bad news or the anticipation of any future event. It is the number one remedy for stage fright and "test amnesia" where the mind goes completely blank and the individual is unable to answer the questions on an examination. Histori-

> *Most commonly you will use Gelsemium when your children or students have test anxiety or stage fright.*

cally, Gelsemium has been used to resolve cowardice on the battlefield and before any difficult challenge or task. It is also the number one remedy for feelings of guilt from overindulgence. Whenever people have devalued their personal standards and thus wounded their own conscience, Gelsemium will quickly remove their blanket of shame and allow them to choose more wisely in the future.

Candidates for the Gelsemium remedy have no appetite or thirst and the symptoms have a slow onset. A sensation of chilliness rises up their spine and there is a dull, heavy ache in the back of the head. Dizziness may also be present.

Key Symptoms Remedied by Gelsemium:

- Chilliness in the spine
- Classic flu symptoms
- Stage fright
- Guilt from overindulgence
- Weakness and collapse

- Lack of appetite or thirst
- Slow onset of symptoms
- Dull, heavy ache in the back of the head
- Dizziness

Most commonly you will use Gelsemium when your children or students have test anxiety or stage fright. This common remedy is usually given at 30c potency and can be found at any health food store that carries homeopathic remedies.

Homeopathic Remedies for Anxiety, Fear and Doubt

Our basic survival instincts trigger powerful surges of vitality that are meant to be used to help us escape from danger. Once these forces are unleashed, their momentum feels unstoppable. Today we no longer need to outrun tigers or leap mountain gorges, and yet our survival instincts still carry the same amount of power required to perform these feats. The modern tiger today dwells in the mind. It appears in the form of mortification, unexpected losses and the fear of the unknown. Regardless of the emotion, your metabolism is at its peak and is prepared to leap the gorge in a single bound. When this tremendous surge of power is not expressed through strenuous physical feats, overwhelming feelings of anxiety and panic inevitably result.

When physical exercise and psychotherapy are unable to wear down these frightful surges, I have found homeopathic remedies to be a godsend. Everyone should know of the homeopathic options for anxiety, fear and doubt. In my experience, there are four remedies that are commonly helpful for these maladies. While the actual list of remedies could be endless, we will review the characteristics of Aconite, Arsenicum album, Calcarea carbonicum and Phosphorous.

ACONITE

Aconite (Aconitum napellus) is famous for resolving anguish and the fear of impending doom. The patient feels that death is close at hand and unavoidable. She may even predict or declare that death will come for her at a specific date and time. Often the Aconite patient has claustrophobia, a fear of earthquakes and a fear of crowded rooms. When a person becomes anxious after a very frightening experience, such as a car accident or a fall down the stairs, this anxiety continues to grow even after the event has passed. The patient is extremely restless and commonly worried about the safety of others. The fear of impending doom is obvious in the patient's facial expression and demeanor of restless haste.

> *Aconite is famous for resolving anguish and the fear of impending doom.*

Key Symptoms Remedied by Aconite:
- Fear of impending doom
- Intense restlessness and agitation
- Prediction of when death will come for them
- Unbearable, frightening pains which alternate with sensations of numbness
- Sudden illness from exposure to extreme cold or extreme heat
- Inconsolable anxiety
- Anxious dreams and nightmares

Aconite given at 30c potency can greatly quell the patient's fears and anxieties. Aconite is one of the most common homeopathic remedies.

Arsenicum Album

Arsenicum album patients are proper, tense and anxious. Like Aconite patients, they have tremendous anxiety and restlessness. However, Arsenicum patients are especially worse after midnight and are constantly seeking reassurance, which they rarely believe. They try to remain in control at all times and, in this state, we see them as perfectionists who have a strong desire for companionship and orderliness. They often fear that they have life-threatening diseases, such as cancer or heart disease, and that they will never recover.

> *Arsenicum album patients are proper, tense, and anxious.*

Key Symptoms Remedied by Arsenicum Album:

- Properness and perfectionism to the extreme
- Tenseness
- Anxiousness
- Restlessness with weakness (desire movement but then discover their weakness)
- Strong desire for orderliness and companionship
- Strong desire to be warm
- Burning pains relieved by warmth
- Appear to be weak, pale and cold, improved by heat

The keynote of Arsenicum is the restlessness and weakness. Arsenicum is also commonly found in health food stores at a 30c potency.

Calcarea Carbonicum

The Calcarea carbonicum patient by nature is solid, sturdy, hardworking and very responsible. He is practical, methodical, and appears physically sturdy and attractive. His Ayurvedic constitution is the most pure form of Kapha, with the tendency toward obesity, possessiveness and anxiety. The fear and anxiety of these patients center on practical issues of security and safety. They may develop fears in regard to money, health, and the performance of their duties (at home and at work). Their anxiety can completely undermine their joyful and robust nature. When these wonderful, hardworking folks become overwhelmed and exhausted, their mind becomes weak and they fear that they will go insane. Their determined, obstinate nature, which made them so reliable when healthy, becomes a huge barrier for the physician attempting to reassure them that they will not go insane. They are obstinate when healthy *and* when anxious.

The fear and anxiety of Calcarea carbonicum patients center on practical issues of security and safety.

When a patient of mine was diagnosed with cancer, she was completely convinced that she would die in the shortest time span possible. Immediately she began to plan financial matters for her children and grandchildren and systematically started to give away her possessions. Her obstinate nature was so convinced that she would die quickly that she could not accept clinical proof showing otherwise. Even after three years of being cancer free, she was still not convinced of her cure. It was only after the fourth year of good health that she finally stopped giving away her possessions and organizing her funeral. Today, thanks to modern medicine and the homeopathic remedy Calcarea carbonicum, she is a healthy and proud grandmother.

Key Traits & Symptoms Remedied by Calcarea Carbonicum:

- Obstinate nature
- Sturdy physically
- Responsible, hardworking, practical
- Anxious, fears concerning money and health

Calcarea carbonicum is a common remedy in your health food store at a 30c potency.

PHOSPHOROUS

The Phosphorous patient opens his heart to everyone and is gullible and suggestible. His unbridled sympathy for everyone, friend and stranger alike, further dilutes his focus and productivity. These individuals appear spacey, diffuse and easily distracted. They startle easily and are easily reassured. Known for their beautiful eyes and facial complexion, their overwhelming kindness makes them easy to like and an easy target for needy, manipulative people. Any thought or idea can trigger their anxiety; likewise, any thought or idea from someone else can resolve their anxiety. Generally, their anxiety is worse from fasting and from too much travel. Their anxiety is greatly reduced by consuming warm, heavy meals and minimizing their excursions.

This type of child has an extremely open, trusting nature, and quickly offers sympathy and love to everyone they meet.

Many years ago, some family friends sent their college-age son to me for help. He had entered a state of openness and gullibility that allowed his girlfriend to dominate his life. Eagerly running at full speed to please his girlfriend, he ignored his duties as son, employee and friend, and soon he became an anxious and confused fellow.

I quickly accepted him into my home for the weekend, knowing that the cure was only 24 or 36 hours away. Our mutual families had known each other for over a decade and the young man, Rob, was willing to accept counsel. His simple treatment program was both Ayurvedic and homeopathic.

Rob was a thick, Kaphic young man who had entered a Vatic (phosphorous-like) state of anxiety. I asked Rob to stay in our guest room in the lower level for 24 hours. I instructed him to not read, write, talk or listen to the radio. This solitude would allow his scattered mind to regroup. I also taught him some simple relaxation exercises. All Rob needed to do was simply pull himself back together by no longer running around trying to please others. Because his constitution was very strong, the correction occurred very quickly. Along with his restriction to this clean and pleasant room, he was given one dose of Phosphorous 200C.

> *The Phosphorous patient opens his heart to everyone and is gullible and suggestible.*

The next morning we saw a miraculous turnaround. His confidence, his clarity, and his practical coping skills were back at his command. His 24 hours of rest and isolation from the duties and opinions of others allowed his system to come back into balance. From his arrival on Friday afternoon until his departure on Sunday afternoon, a great transformation had occurred, due simply to the power of homeopathic Phosphorous and a proper understanding of his Ayurvedic nature.

Key Traits & Symptoms Remedied by Phosphorous:

- Gullibility
- A tendency to be easily reassured by others
- A need to please others

Phosphorus is commonly found in health food stores at a 30c potency.

STAPHYSAGRIA

For over 20 years the most commonly used remedy in my medical practice has been one that treats suppressed anger and the various ailments that arise from this suppression. I see women going through divorces where their life and social status have been devastated. In a sad form of irony, it seems that women who saw their physical beauty as their strongest social acclaim suffered from outbreaks of bright red, dry eczema on their forehead and eyebrows during these times of stress and anger. The more they suppress their rage and mortification, the brighter and larger the rash becomes. Likewise, any other ailment that begins with a history of suppressed anger and low self-esteem requires us to consider this remedy.

Initially these patients appear sweet and passive in nature. Gradually they reveal a long history of grief and degrading situations. They have responded to these events with shame and guilt, while anger and defiance would be a healthy reaction. Often, they have allowed themselves to be dominated for many years. When Staphysagria

> *Initially Staphysagria patients appear sweet and passive in nature. Gradually they reveal a long history of grief and degrading situations.*

helps them rally their courage and mental clarity, I commonly see such meek, humiliated people make a huge and healthy transformation. Staphysagria is known for improving one's self-esteem. And this remedy isn't just relegated to dominated spouses. Whenever a person presents a history of humiliation and suppression from an older sibling or parent, Staphysagria should be carefully considered.

Key Traits & Symptoms Remedied by Staphysagria:
- History of humiliation and degrading experiences
- Suppressed anger
- Sweetness and passivity
- Shame and guilt about sexuality

Because this remedy usually deals with a deep level of suppression, 200c is commonly the starting dose. Therefore, you will usually have to visit a homeopathic pharmacy.

CLINICAL STUDIES

Due to the infinitesimal doses involved in homeopathic remedy production, the modern medical community wonders if the success of homeopathic care is due to the placebo effect. However, many double-blind clinical trials have validated the effectiveness of homeopathy on a broad range of illnesses.

One such study was done in 1994 by the Department of Epidemiology at the University of Washington in Seattle. It performed a clinical trial on children stricken with diarrhea in Nicaragua. This double-blind placebo-controlled trial found that "individualized homeopathic treatment decreases the duration of diarrhea and number of stools in children with acute childhood diarrhea."[18]

Another study, published in the Lancet in 1986, sought to discover whether homeopathy was effective in the treatment of allergies and hay fever. That study found that, "patients using homeopathy showed greater improvement in symptoms than those on placebo."[19]

A third study, published in the British Journal of Homeopathy, also found that homeopathy was helpful for children with attention deficit disorder (ADD or ADHD). This study compared the effectiveness of methylphenidate (Ritalin) to homeopathic care. The findings were dramatic – "The reported results of homeopathic treatment appear to be similar to the effects of MPD (Ritalin)."[20] This landmark study dramatically changed the lives of many parents and children when they discovered that they could switch away from a powerful medication to a completely safe, non-toxic homeopathic remedy.

There are many more studies that show the efficacy of homeopathy. There have been some poorly constructed studies that have attempted to discredit homeopathy by giving the same homeopathic remedy to every member in the study. However, this is not how homeopathy works – the remedy must be carefully chosen for each individual. As more clinical studies, that are properly conducted, show the benefits of homeopathy, it will continue to grow in popularity.

> *The physician of the future will skillfully integrate homeopathic medicine into his/her repertoire alongside Ayurvedic therapies, surgery, diet therapies, prescription drugs and herbal therapies.*

HOMEOPATHY: THE MEDICINE OF THE FUTURE

In the past few pages I have shared with you some homeopathic solutions for those very difficult situations when hope seems lost. Whether you're experiencing profound sadness from the loss of a loved one, or deep anger from past actions, homeopathic remedies offer you a safe and natural way to resolve your torment.

Homeopathy is a system of medicine that has been helping people break these kinds of longstanding habits of self-condemnation and doubt for more than 200 years; but only in the past 50 years has homeopathy seen a resurgence in the United States. This resurgence will continue as a new model of patient care evolves. It is the simplicity, safety, and quality of homeopathy that makes it so appealing today.

Gone will be the days of pushing through 12 patients an hour and prescribing "cookie cutter" solutions for each patient. Instead, the physicians will aim to understand their patients on all levels, leading to improved patient care and superior results. Furthermore, when the physician takes the time to understand the patient on a deeper level, then the patient benefits from feeling understood. The physician benefits from finding the correct homeopathic remedy. In an age when antibiotics are becoming ineffective and diseases are more easily transmitted, homeopathy offers great hope for the future. The physician of the future will skillfully integrate homeopathic medicine into his/her repertoire alongside Ayurvedic therapies, surgery, diet therapies, prescription drugs and herbal therapies.

CHAPTER SUMMARY

- *Homeopathy often helps people overcome physical and psychological problems when other therapies have failed and the problem seems impossible to overcome.*

- *Homeopathic medicines have the unique ability to help you get through difficult situations. Sometimes, when you get stuck in a bout of sadness and grief, homeopathy can help release pent-up feelings that you have suppressed and bring you back to a state of happiness.*

- *In an age when antibiotics are becoming ineffective and diseases are more easily transmitted, homeopathy offers great hope for the future.*

Chapter

Sleep, Rest and Relaxation

I t had been a very long day at the office for me. And now an overwhelmed mother was expounding on her lists of grievances in regards to her 8-year-old son; the little boy sitting next to her. His sadness pulled him deeper into his chair as he listened to his mother's itemized complaints. He didn't flinch, he just drooped. Item number five was how restless he was – constantly in motion, unable to sit still.

For ages, parents have complained to me about how restless their children are, but on that late afternoon I heard "restless" in a completely new way. Restless. "Why does he get *less rest* than your other children?" I blurted it out. I was questioning myself as well as the boy's mother. At that moment, even I didn't really know what I meant.

I knew how irritable I became when I was overly tired. If I did not get enough rest I would probably be bouncing off the walls. Maybe that was little Curt's problem also? If an 8-year-old is not well rested, could he be expressing his loss in aimless motions and mutterings? I looked up. Curt's mom was staring at me with her jaw open. I had either sounded ridiculous or stumbled across a major clue. As our eyes met, she started nodding in agreement.

Less rest – exactly! That must be it. Ever since Curt's little brother had started whining at night, Curt had been more restless. Having a baby brother teething in the same bedroom may have been the very cause of Curt not getting enough rest. They moved him to his older sister's bedroom and within three days his restlessness had diminished by 75 percent, according to the follow-up email from his mother.

We all need rest. If you're lucky, sleep is restful; but for most of us, sleep is rarely restful. I ask my patients questions like: Do you wake up feeling dull and groggy? Do you feel stressed and rushed all day because, once again, you overslept? Do you feel that no matter how much sleep you get, it's never enough? This is not how sleep is supposed to feel. If that is your experience, then something needs to change. I am going to show you how and why your sleep habits may need improvement.

At bedtime, many of my patients get dragged into unconsciousness. They go to bed so tired that they have no control over the experience and quality of their sleep. They

> *To be happy and healthy, you have to stop being a victim to your dietary habits, your breathing patterns and your sleeping patterns.*

collapse into their beds, only to wake hours later feeling like a slave to their sleep habits. To be happy and healthy, you have to stop being a victim to your dietary habits, your breathing patterns and your sleep patterns. These activities are deeply embedded but they can be drastically modified for the better. Understanding both the modern scientific and Ayurvedic suggestions for sleep will liberate you from the tormenting dullness and grogginess that poor sleep produces.

When I talk to audiences today, I always incorporate the topic of sleep. This is because we have forgotten how to truly rest. I always ask my listeners if they have ever slept eight hours and woken up exhausted. No matter where I am, the hands fly up. "What were you doing for those eight hours?" I ask them. They are not exactly sure how those hours were spent – all they know is that they were not restful. This universal experience of sleep shows that there must be a difference between sleep and rest – otherwise sleeping eight hours would always leave you feeling rested.

REST AND RELAXATION – THE PRELUDE TO SLEEP

I inform my audiences that it is important to practice resting and relaxation on a daily basis. The ultimate form of stress management is the discovery that you are more powerful and more creative than you thought. This discovery, this revelation, is only possible through cleansing the doors of perception that stand between you, your mind and your world. Rest and relaxation are cleansing techniques that will lead to this grand discovery. Such techniques can have a profound impact on your life and your relationships.

> *Rest and relaxation are cleansing techniques that can have a profound impact on your life and your relationships.*

Rest is a cleansing technique that removes dullness and inertia. Relaxation is also a cleansing technique, but it is designed to remove restlessness and anxiety. If the body is busy digesting food or if your mind is busy digesting thoughts or sounds (like music, television or other background noise), then you are not cleansing yourself, but rather nourishing yourself. Both music and food require the attention and energy of your mind and body to be processed, but it is not conducive to an inward unveiling of your higher qualities. Thus, it seems logical that *relaxation music* limits your level of relaxation to a pleasant state of sensory satisfaction. But to discover your finest qualities deep within you, you will need to slowly and gently cleanse away the layers of restlessness from your mind and nervous system. This is best done in silence. Relaxation is an active part of the self-transformation process. You will come in touch with the bright shiny parts of your personality and discover yourself through the daily practice of relaxation.

Any effective relaxation and rest technique must be cleansing. Cleansing is brought about by fresh air, fresh water and the fire of your body's metabolism. You can take dullness and restlessness and blow it away, wash it away or burn it away. Blowing refers to breathing techniques; washing refers to clean water in the form of beverages and bathing; and burning refers to the friction from the movement of your skeletal muscles, lungs, abdomen and respiratory diaphragm. You can regain your vigor in 7-16 minutes with these techniques in almost any location. I call this the 'real power nap.' All you need is proper instruction and a quiet, stable environment where you can close your eyes. Being able to lay comfortably flat on your back is optimal. If you have the luxury of more time and floor space, then you can achieve even deeper states of relaxation and rest.

Before we advance to the 'power nap' technique, I would like to help you build a firm foundation with the basic breathing techniques to create balance and harmony in your life. There are four prerequisites (diaphragmatic breathing, alternate nostril breathing, the 61 Point Relaxation Exercise and the Advanced Relaxation technique) that will allow you to enter the realm of the real power nap and yoga nidra discussed in the next chapter.

RELAXATION

Removing anxiety and restlessness from your mind and body is as simple as breathing through your nose. All you need to do is focus on the sensations of coolness and warmth at the tip of your nose and quickly the mind will become quiet and the body will relax.

The first three methods -- diaphragmatic breathing, alternate nostril breathing and the 61 Point Relaxation Exercise -- were explained in detail in my earlier book, **Happiness: The Real Medicine and How It Works.** I have excerpted the details for you here.

Quieting the Mind with Diaphragmatic Breathing

Joining the mind with breath is a powerful way to quiet the mind. Start by getting your breath to flow only through your nose in a quiet, serene manner. Allow your upper chest and shoulders to stay quiet and still, as the abdomen expands during inhalation and then gently exhale collapsing your abdomen and upper chest. This motion in the abdomen will create a profound sense of peace and relaxation. The movement of the respiratory diaphragm (which separates the chest cavity from the abdomen) stimulates the vagus nerve. This nerve is the tenth cranial nerve and has a parasympathetic action on the entire body. This action calms and cleanses. Breathing diaphragmatically will activate the vagus nerve and a sense of relaxation will result.

When you bring the mind to the tip of the nose, right inside the nose, on the wall that divides the two nostrils, notice the temperature of the air as it enters and leaves the body. Commonly, room temperature is around 70 degrees Fahrenheit and the body maintains a core temperature around 98 degrees.

Because of this 28 degree difference in temperatures, notice that during inhalation a sense of coolness plays at the tip of the nose. When the air is inside your lungs, the body will heat it up. Therefore, during exhalation, the air will feel slightly warmer at the tip of the nose as it flows out of the body. Take a few minutes right now to experience this.

Let your abdomen rise and fall with each breath. Notice how the restlessness, itchiness, and tension melt away as you continue to focus on your breath.

Eliminate any pause between inhalation and exhalation as your breath becomes smooth, slow, continuous, and quiet. Make a smooth transition between inhalation and exhalation. Bring your awareness to the tip of your nose so you can feel the slight sensation of coolness every time you inhale and the faint sensation of warmth on exhalation. Maintain your awareness of the sensation of coolness during inhalation and warmth during exhalation.

Allow the breath to slow down. Slow, serene breathing will increase your capacity to focus on the object of your meditation (the sensations inside the tip of your nose). It is very important to stay within your comfortable capacity. Do not strain the breath. Before concluding the practice, observe what has happened to your mind and body during this time.[21]

Alternate Nostril Breathing (Nadi Shodhana)

Alternate nostril breathing is a technique designed to balance both hemispheres of the brain, calm the nervous system, and deeply relax muscular tension throughout your body. According to yoga science and modern day research, when air flows through the right nostril, it innervates the sympathetic nervous system. Likewise, when air flows through the left nostril, the parasympathetic nervous system is activated. The balancing effect of alternate nostril breathing re-energizes your body's metabolism and improves your concentration. It is one of the most profound and important techniques for rejuvenation, relaxation, and for learning more advanced yogic practices.

Alternate nostril breathing is based upon the physiology of the nose: the two nostrils and the turbinates inside them. The role of the nose in general is to warm, moisten, and cleanse the air you breath in. There are three turbinates in each of your nostrils; they have a shape similar to a jet engine turbine. These turbinates swell with blood, increase in size, and then shrink back to normal size in a cyclic manner. The turbinates also have the ability to change the subtle electrical charge of flowing air with the very fine hairs that line the nostril cavity.

When engaged in alternate nostril breathing, you are controlling this otherwise natural, cyclic function that happens 24 hours a day, 7 days a week. Throughout the 24-hour cycle, one nostril is always more open to air flow. This nostril is called the active nostril. The other nostril, called the passive nostril, is more closed to airflow due to the swelling of the turbinates. Every 90-120 minutes, the dominance of the openings of the nostrils switch. If right now you can breathe more freely through your right nostril, in about two hours, you will be able to breathe more freely through the other nostril. This is called an "ultradian rhythm" – a process which repeats itself in a cycle shorter than 24 hours.

If the air flowing through your nostrils is perfectly even, that means you are right in that center phase as the airflow is switching from one nostril to the other. Having both nostrils completely equal and open is a very important time. In yoga science, that is called *sushumna*, a Sanskrit word meaning joyous, joyous mind. It refers to an experiential and neurobiological fact. When both of your nostrils are even and open, you will notice that your mind is very happy and content.

When breathing during the time period of sushumna, you will more easily experience a joyous, joyous mind. The end result of alternate nostril breathing is sushumna. This is very helpful for meditators who first practice alternate nostril breathing and achieve sushumna, the joyous, content state of the mind. Once the mind is content and joyous, you can more easily meditate.

Alternate nostril breathing has a history of therapeutic use in the yoga tradition dating back thousands of years. This technique has been used to assist with stress management, chronic diseases, and a myriad of psychological disorders. In this next section, we will explore the three basic techniques that yoga science teaches for practicing alternate nostril breathing.

There are three ways to practice alternate nostril breathing. The consistent characteristic of all styles is that they involve breathing for a specific number of times through one nostril, switching to the opposite nostril, and then breathing through both nostrils.

One way of practicing alternate nostril breathing is to inhale through the right nostril and exhale through the left nostril. We can continue in this manner, inhaling right and exhaling left, for three times and then change to inhaling through the left and exhaling through the right for three times. The final step in this style of alternate nostril breathing is to breathe through both nostrils for three times. This total of nine breaths is referred to as one "round" or "set" of alternate nostril breathing, and very often you would perform three rounds in one sitting.

A second style of alternate nostril breathing is inhaling through the right nostril, exhaling through the left nostril, then inhaling through the left, and exhaling through the right. This series is usually practiced three times to constitute one "set" or "round." Three sets comprise the practice.

A third style is exhaling and inhaling through the right nostril three times concluding with an exhale, then inhaling and exhaling through the left nostril three times. Finally, inhale and exhale for three times through both nostrils. This is also considered one "set."

❀   ❀   ❀

Alternate nostril breathing has a profound ability to completely balance every aspect of the mind, the body, and the breath. Medical research shows that just ten minutes of alternate nostril breathing can dramatically affect brain waves in a positive manner.

Commonly, three sets of alternate nostril breathing are practiced once or twice a day. If you have the ability to do more than three sets, the practice can be even more profound. Some people practice alternate nostril breathing based upon time rather than the number of sets. However, it is important to always finish the set, with the last three breaths through both nostrils.

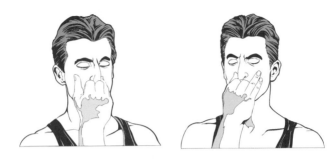

ALTERNATE NOSTRIL BREATHING

Let's go through the actual practice of alternate nostril breathing. If possible, it is best to use the right thumb and right ring finger to close off the nostrils. The right thumb is used to close off the right nostril, and the right ring finger is used to close off the left nostril. We will go through three complete sets of alternate nostril breathing. Although there are several ways to practice alternate nostril breathing, for most beginners, the easiest way is to focus on one nostril for three breaths, the other nostril for three breaths, and then both nostrils for three breaths.

• Begin by closing your right nostril with your right thumb. Exhale smoothly and slowly, quietly and diaphragmatically. Don't overextend your breath or make the breath too quick.

• Now inhale. Concentrate on your left nostril breathing in and out for three times. Try to make the flow of the breath continuous so as soon as you are done inhaling, you begin exhaling.

• As soon as you are done exhaling, begin inhaling. Then close your left nostril with your right ring finger and repeat the process.

• Next, breathe through both nostrils for three breaths. You have now completed your first set of the nine breaths. Please continue alternate nostril breathing for two more sets.

Start your regular practice by finding a little bit of time away from the noises of the day when you can sit still for five or ten minutes. Start to work with your breath and allow your head, neck, and trunk to be straight. The more you practice alternate nostril breathing, the more your understanding will deepen. You may want to contact a teacher for further advancement. There are many levels to alternate nostril breathing as you progress down the path of self-transformation.[22]

An Introduction to 61 Points

The 61-Point Relaxation exercise is a more advanced technique that requires floor space to lay down and about 10-15 minutes of your time. The 61-Point Relaxation exercise is one of the most profound methods of rejuvenation. It is actually much more than a relaxation exercise. It is considered an advanced practice because it means that the student by this time has already learned how to breathe diaphragmatically and has learned how to practice some form of systematic relaxation. An experienced practitioner of systematic relaxation has learned how to lay down and relax the body without falling asleep. Similarly, most advanced practices require you to have the ability to stay awake when doing something more subtle, more inward.

The posture for 61-Points is called the corpse pose*, or *shivasana*, in which you lay down on your back with your palms toward the sky and your feet as wide as your shoulders. Put a little pillow under your head which will prevent pressure in your esophagus. You have a constant air bubble in your stomach, and when you are practicing deep relaxation, the sphincter that closes the junction between the esophagus and

the stomach relaxes. If it relaxes, the air bubble in the stomach could come up and put subtle pressure in your esophagus.
To keep the esophagus closed, you must raise the head up
about an inch or two. Thus, the purpose of the pillow is not
for the comfort of your head but rather to raise the head. In
the beginning of learning this exercise, this is not a big deal,
but later on, as you experience deeper and deeper states of
relaxation, you should practice 61-Points with a pillow.

When laying in the corpse pose, you should have a light
blanket covering you, so that other air currents do not affect
the current of the mind as it travels through the body. Protect
yourself from noises -- make sure the telephones are off, and
do not answer the doorbell. If your spouse is practicing with
you, and you have small children, I recommend that one of
you keep an eye on the kids while the other one does 61-
Points and then switch.

Once you have acquired the experience of relaxation, then
61-Points really helps deepen that experience. You will be
using your mental awareness to travel through 61 different
points throughout the body. At each point, you will bring
your mental awareness there. To make sure both the right
(creativity and colors) and left (analytical and numbers)
hemispheres of the brain are involved at each point, visualize a blue dot and also the number of that dot. The blue
color represents a deep form of relaxation. Of all the colors in
the mind, visualizing blue is the most relaxing. These points
are called *marma sthanas*, meaning a delicate intersection or
place. There are several types of *marma* points. In 61-Points,
the marma points are visualized as being blue because they
have to do with cleansing, rejuvenation, and relaxation. As

* The corpse pose is illustrated in Chapter 5.

you travel through your body, you may encounter a marma point that causes your body to flinch or twitch. This experience is the release of tension. You may also encounter points of dullness – causing you to forget what you are doing or causing you to briefly fall asleep. Don't be disappointed when these things happen. Falling asleep is cleansing.

The 61 Points

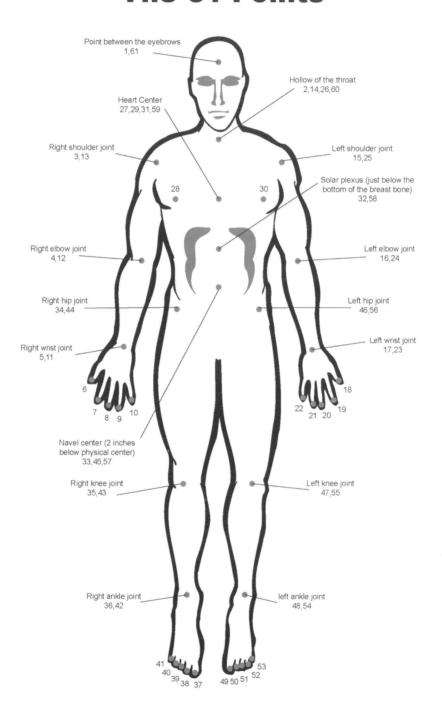

Point between the eyebrows
1,61

Hollow of the throat
2,14,26,60

Heart Center
27,29,31,59

Right shoulder joint
3,13

Left shoulder joint
15,25

Solar plexus (just below the
bottom of the breast bone)
32,58

28

30

Right elbow joint
4,12

Left elbow joint
16,24

Right hip joint
34,44

Left hip joint
46,56

Right wrist joint
5,11

Left wrist joint
17,23

6

18

7

10

8 9

22

19

21 20

Navel center (2 inches
below physical center)
33,45,57

Right knee joint
35,43

Left knee joint
47,55

Right ankle joint
36,42

left ankle joint
48,54

41

53

40

39

52

38 37

49 50 51

THE 61-POINT RELAXATION EXERCISE

Use the chart to learn the location of each point before beginning this exercise. Lay down in the corpse pose as described above and begin your relaxation exercise. Gently bring your awareness to each point and visualize the number at each location along with a blue dot the size of a marble. Travel slowly to each point as you follow them in numerical order.

1- Point between the eyebrows

2- Hollow of the throat

3- Right shoulder joint

4- Right elbow joint

5- The right wrist joint

6- Tip of the right thumb

7- Tip of the right index finger

8- Tip of the right middle finger

9- Tip of the right fourth finger (ring finger)

10- Tip of the right small finger

11- The right wrist joint

12- Right elbow joint

13- Right shoulder joint

14- Hollow of the throat

15- Left shoulder joint

16- Left elbow joint

17- The left wrist joint

18- Tip of the left thumb

19- Tip of the left index finger

20- Tip of the left middle finger

21- Tip of the left fourth finger (ring finger)

22- Tip of the left small finger

23- The left wrist joint

24- Left elbow joint

25- Left shoulder joint

26- Hollow of the throat

27- Heart center

28- Right nipple

29- Heart center

30- Left nipple

31- Heart center

32- Solar plexus (just below the bottom of the breast bone)

33- Navel center (2 inches below the physical navel)

34- Right hip joint

35- Right knee joint

36- Right ankle joint

37- Tip of the right big toe

38- Tip of the right second toe

39- Tip of the right third toe

40- Tip of the right fourth toe

41- Tip of the right small toe

42- Right ankle joint

43- Right knee joint

44- Right hip joint

45- Navel center (2 inches below the physical navel)

46- Left hip joint

47- Left knee joint

48- Left ankle joint

49- Tip of the left big toe

50- Tip of the left second toe

51- Tip of the left third toe

52- Tip of the left fourth toe

53- Tip of the left small toe

54- Left ankle joint

55- Left knee joint

56- Left hip joint

57- Navel center (2 inches below the physical navel)

58- Solar plexus

59- Heart center

60- Hollow of the throat

61- Center between the eyebrows

This was excerpted from Happiness: The Real Medicine and How It Works, pages 77-81, 108.

These three methods – diaphragmatic breathing, alternate nostril breathing, and the 61 Point Relaxation exercise – are for relaxation. They remove restlessness and anxiety from your mind and body. Once you have mastered these techniques, you can move forward to resting techniques that remove dullness and fatigue from your mind and body.

You will begin with learning advanced relaxation, a profound method to provide you with deep rest and an enhanced ability for self-understanding. This advanced relaxation technique can create more space in even the busiest day. Once you know the value of relaxation, it is time to learn another technique that is considered to be more profound than the 61-Point Relaxation exercise. Swami Rama stated that there is no exercise better than this one to alleviate stress.

In Swami Rama's famous text on this practice, *Path of Fire and Light, Volume Two,* he claimed that through this advanced relaxation practice, blood sugars have been seen to decrease by 25 percent and high blood pressure readings have improved. Forty-one cases of insomnia were completely cured in seven days with this exercise. While it is known to resolve insomnia, relaxation exercises are not to be used to fall asleep. This is an important point. Rather, sleep will become easier to achieve because your tension and anxiety will be removed.

Advanced relaxation is also helpful for pain syndromes and removing musculo-skeletal tension.

THE PRELUDE TO ADVANCED RELAXATION

Practice in a room that can be dark and quiet. You need to be protected from noises and interruptions during the 15 or 20 minutes needed for this practice. Lay on the floor in the corpse pose with a small pillow under your head. When you elevate your head by 1-2 inches, it will prevent the gases in your stomach from rising up and disturbing your heart by creating a block at the base of your esophagus.

Cover your entire body, except for your head and neck, with a light blanket that will protect you from chills and drafts. Close your eyes and, if necessary, cover your eyes with a soft cloth to ensure complete darkness. In the corpse pose, extend your arms 16 inches away from your body and have your palms facing the ceiling. Make sure that your legs are wider than your shoulders.

In this exercise, the mind and breath travel together throughout the body. You will be inhaling and exhaling to specific areas within your body. It will be easy to visualize these places. This exercise will expand the flow of prana (energy) and vitality throughout your body, creating more space in the subtle and experiential realms. Eliminate any noise, pauses or jerking in the breath, let the mind and breath flow together. Nasal diaphragmatic breathing is used the entire time.

THE PRACTICE OF ADVANCED RELAXATION

Begin this relaxation practice by breathing diaphragmatically through your nose five times – five complete exhalations and five inhalations. Allow your abdomen to expand on inhalation and gently contract on exhalation. Your mind (mental awareness) and your breath will flow together as you inwardly travel throughout your body during this technique.

THE INWARD JOURNEY OF ADVANCED RELAXATION

The path of yoga is an inward journey. The journey is both a metaphor and a reality. In this exercise you will be enjoining your mental awareness and the pranic aspect of your breath to travel within your body. Initially, this may seem like a fantasy or a new use of your imagination, but in reality you will be learning to literally travel through your body. Once this skill is developed, your inner vision will become quite profound and may be used as a diagnostic tool for the skilled practitioner.

Thousands of years ago, the adepts of yoga were able to accurately diagram the neuropathways of the body through their power of introspection. Their 'inner vision' was more accurate and profound in understanding the body's metabolism than what modern medicine has discovered through the dissection of a corpse.

The technique of inward traveling for the advanced relaxation sequence is quite simple. Allow your breath and mental awareness to flow together in the sequence written in the text and illustrated in the diagram. Keep your awareness in the central core of your physical body. The breath is not to travel along the surface of the body but rather through the center of your body. For example, as your mind and breath travel during exhalation from the crown of your head to your toes, keep them flowing in the innermost core of your physical body.

Exhalation begins at the crown of the head and flows toward the feet. Inhalation always concludes at the crown of the head. No matter from where in the body your inhalation begins, you always continue inhaling until you reach the crown of the head and then stop.

The Advanced Relaxation Sequence

Phase One

Exhale from the crown of your head down to your toes. Inhale from your toes through your ankles, knees, hip joints, spinal column, coming back to the crown of your head for ten full breaths.

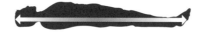

Phase Two

Exhale from the crown of your head to the ankles and inhale back to the crown of the head for ten complete breaths.

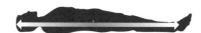

Phase Three

Exhale from the crown of your head to the knees and inhale back up to the crown of the head for five full breaths.

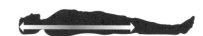

Phase Four

Exhale from the crown of your head to the bottom of your torso (your perineum) and inhale from the perineum to the crown of your head for five full breaths.

Phase Five

Exhale from the crown of your head to your navel center (the solar plexus), and inhale from the solar plexus to the crown of your head for five full breaths.

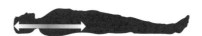

Phase Six

Exhale from the crown of your head to your heart center in the middle of your chest, and inhale from your heart center to the crown of your head for five full breaths.

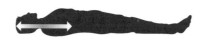

Phase Seven

Exhale from the crown of your head to the throat, and inhale from the throat to the crown of your head for five full breaths.

Phase Eight

Exhale from the crown of your head to the bridge between the nostrils, and inhale from the bridge between the nostrils to the crown of your head for five full breaths.

Phase Nine

Let your mind and conciousness pay attention to the inhalation and exhalation flowing between the nostrils and the space between the two eyebrows. Let the mind and breath flow between these two points for ten to twenty-five complete breaths.

Now, reverse the practice.

The first phase of this exercise begins upon completing the first five breaths. Bring your awareness to the top of your head and exhale from the crown of your head down to your toes. On exhale, empty yourself and expel all of your toxins, fatigues, stress and strains. On inhale, know that you are inhaling energy from the atmosphere. Inhale from your toes through your ankles, knees, hip joints, spinal column, coming back to the crown of the head. Do not allow the breath to pause or stop. Let the mind and breath flow together exhaling toward the toes, inhaling up to the crown of the head for 10 full breaths. Please note that this exercise begins with an exhalation and ends on the 10th inhalation. Thus you enter the second phase of the exercise with an exhalation.

The second phase is to exhale from the crown of the head to the ankles and inhale back up to the crown of the head for 10 complete breaths. Next, phase three begins on exhale from the crown of the head to the knees and inhaling from the knees to the crown of the head for 5 full breaths. In phase four, you exhale from your crown to the bottom of your torso -- your perineum -- and inhale from the perineum to the crown of your head for five full breaths.

In phase five, you exhale from your crown to your navel center (the solar plexus), and inhale from the solar plexus to the crown of your head for five full breaths. In phase six, you exhale from your crown to the heart center in the middle of your chest, and inhale from the heart center to the crown of your head for five full breaths. In phase seven, you exhale from your crown to the throat, and inhale from the throat to the crown of your head for five full breaths.

In phase eight, you exhale from your crown to the bridge between the two nostrils, and inhale from the bridge between the nostrils to the crown of your head for five full breaths. During this phase your breath should become very fine and short. Even the motion of your lungs will have a shorter rhythm. The focal point is where the nasal septum joins the face directly above the upper lip. This spot is located at the junction between two nostrils on the face and not on the nose -- technically, the junction between the philtrum and the septum.

In phase nine, the final phase, let your mind and consciousness pay attention to the inhalation and exhalation flowing between the two nostrils and the space between the two eyebrows. Let the mind and breath flow between these two points for 10-25 complete breaths.

At this point, you start to reverse the practice. You will always start each new breathing pattern with an exhalation – as if to purge yourself of the old and exhausted before you can be renewed with fresh pranic energy. You will breathe for five complete breaths at each point until you reach the lower areas of your body where you will breath for 10 full breaths. You will begin the reversal of this exercise by exhaling from the crown of your head to the center of the nostrils for five full breaths. Next, exhale to your throat for five breaths. Next, exhale from your crown to your heart center for five breaths. Next, exhale from your crown to your solar plexus and back for five breaths. Next, exhale from the crown of your head to your perineum at the base of your torso for five breaths. Next, exhale from the crown of your head to your knee joints for five breaths. Next, exhale from the crown of your head to your ankles for 10 breaths. Finally, exhale from the crown of your head to your toes for 10 breaths. This concludes this exercise.

You are returning from a state of deep relaxation, please go slowly as you re-awaken your body. While remaining in the corpse pose, start to gently wiggle your fingers and toes. Bring your hands together and rub your palms vigorously to heat them up. Then gently place your warm palms over your eyes. Gradually let your eyes open into the darkness of the palms, keeping the eyes open as you gently remove your hands. Bring both knees to the chest and gently rock the knees and back from side to side. Then gently roll to your left side with the knees curled toward the chest and lie there for 30-60 seconds. During this phase of re-awakening your body, this position allows all the essential fluids to return to the region of your heart as you prepare to rise up and re-start your day. Gently use both arms to push yourself up into a seated position and return to your duties of the day.

*You can download this instruction sheet along with a graphic for **Advanced Relaxation** at www.AliveandHealthy.com.*

The regular practice of these relaxation techniques will benefit you, your family and your community. As you experience the personal benefits of being free from worry and doubt, it is natural to wonder about the possibilities of how the science of sleep could further transform your life. You are ready to explore the concepts of yoga nidra.

CHAPTER SUMMARY

- *Rest and relaxation exercises are cleansing techniques. Rest removes dullness and inertia while relaxation removes restlessness and anxiety.*

- *Rest and relaxation are important prerequisites to good sleep. If you go to sleep anxious and restless, your quality of sleep will suffer.*

ACTION ITEMS

- *Practice one full round of alternate nostril breathing each day for 11 days and observe the effect.*

- *Practice the 61-point relaxation exercise daily until you can complete the exercise regularly without falling asleep.*

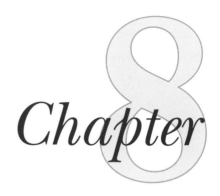

Chapter 8

Yoga Nidra:
The Science of Yogic Sleep

L earning and practicing relaxation techniques are the experiential prerequisites to learning about sleep and rest. Building on what you have learned in the previous chapter, we are now going to explore the relationship between sleep, sleep cycles, rest and a yoga technique called yoga nidra (yogic sleep). You are going to learn how to have better sleep than ever before. This skill has countless benefits, both psychologically and practically. When you are able to wake up feeling refreshed and alert, happiness will naturally come easier. When you have the ability to attain deep rest and therefore can sleep less, you will have more time for your life and you will feel less stressed.

Rest and relaxation are the prelude to sleep. With the dullness and worries of the day removed, you can go to sleep easily and reap full benefits from your time asleep. To learn the science of sleep, you must first practice the skills of resting and relaxation. Rest is achieved by using a technique to cleanse and clear away dullness and inertia.

Sleepiness is that dullness. Yoga science recommends specific breathing techniques to remove tiredness and dullness. These methods provide rest and renewal to your mind and body.

Relaxation is achieved by using a technique to cleanse and clear away anxiety and restlessness. Any technique that offers relaxation and rest must be a cleansing technique.

When dullness and inertia take the wind out of your sails, leaving you motionless at your desk, you know you need help to get through your day. Instead of running for coffee or a cigarette, this is the moment that resting techniques can bring you back to life. There have been way too many moments when my personal levels of fatigue were so high that I feared I might fall asleep at my own seminar. When I find myself so exhausted that gravity seems to have doubled its strength, I quicken my pace so that I can last until the next 15-minute intermission.

All you need is 7-16 minutes to rest so deeply that you can get your wind back. Your clarity and enthusiasm will be fully charged in just a few minutes. Thanks to this technique, the long days of my seminars never defeat me. I call it the 'real power nap.'

REST AND THE REAL POWER NAP

Here is the theory behind this technique. Your enthusiasm and attention span can become dull from the inability to process incoming substances and information. Holistically, good digestion means that you are able to digest food and beverages, as well as information and sensory stimulation. Feeling heavy and dull in the head can be caused by your diet, by a lack of exercise or by a sensory overload of information and emotions. Likewise, the digestive fire in your abdomen – specifically the region of your solar plexus – can be stimulated by breathing diaphragmatically in a slow, strong continuous manner. As your lungs and abdomen expand and contract, like a gentle bellows, the pranic power within you starts to rebuild. In 7 – 16 minutes, you will start to feel alert and vital again.

The internal friction of your respiratory diaphragm will create enough heat to burn away the dullness and inertia that makes you sleepy and slow. The following technique can be performed in a chair, but once again, laying supine on the floor is optimal.

Here is the technique. Imagine that you are in a situation where sleepiness is trying to control you and becoming drowsy is completely unacceptable. Let us also agree that you are in reasonably good health and you are usually well rested. If your sleepiness is associated with driving a vehicle, you must stop and rest. This is not the time to use these techniques for the very first time. Master the following system and then with full agility you can apply it in your life as you see reasonable and safe.

First, get up and move around. Swing your arms, do some toe touches, and breathe deeply. Drink a couple of glasses of clean water. Find a quiet place where you can lay down for a few minutes without being interrupted. Lay in the corpse pose* and use a small pillow under your head. Breathe through your nose in a smooth, slow, continuous fashion. Allow your abdomen to rise with each inhalation and fall with every exhalation.

The essence of this exercise is to increase the pranic pressure and digestive fire in your solar plexus. This process will remove dullness from both your mind and body. It is simple to do: breathe with a feeling of strength and sturdiness in your breath. Exaggerate the movements of your abdomen as you breathe. Visualize fire filling your entire abdominal cavity and see every inhalation fanning the flames of this fire.

As the visualization of fire becomes natural, relax your intensity and let the process become automatic. Continue to lay in a comfortable fashion and observe the flow of your breath and the motion of your abdomen. Let the floor completely support your body.

* The corpse pose is illustrated in Chapter 5.

There is a secondary benefit to this practice when you add one final component – the time factor. Ask your mind to let you rest for the 7–16 minute duration of this practice and to, more importantly, have your mind gently alert you when the time is completed. Choose a precise number of minutes and direct your mind to awaken you at the end of that time. Your mind is

> *Your mind is your servant and your best friend.*

your servant and your best friend when such qualities are cultivated. Trusting your mind to watch over you and to alert you on schedule is a very fine way to develop a powerful relationship with your mind. Make your mind reliable. As the two of you become best friends, wonderful things can happen.

The Power of Napping

Napping is often taken as a sign of laziness. However, will you get more done if you struggle through hours of work when you are exhausted, or if you opt to take a nap and return to work refreshed and enthusiastic? Throughout history, many famously productive people have chosen the latter, so if you would too, you are in good company. Leonardo Da Vinci, Thomas Edison, Albert Einstein, Winston Churchill, Johannes Brahms, Buckminster Fuller, Salvador Dali and many others all used napping to increase their productivity in their work.[23]

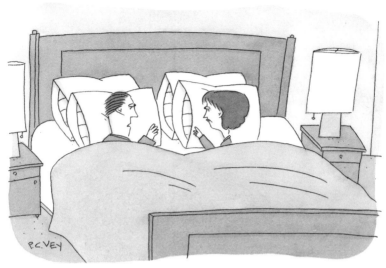

*"I just don't feel right unless I get my normal eight hours
of semiconscious drifting in and out of sleep."*

THE ANATOMY OF SLEEP

Both modern science and the science of Ayurveda agree that you
can learn to sleep more efficiently and more skillfully. Modern scientific studies show that sleeping too long can leave you feeling lethargic. Likewise, Ayurveda stresses the importance of waking up
on time, specifically before sunrise. Modern science has shown the
importance of not eating immediately before bedtime. Ayurveda
concurs and encourages a 12-hour fast between 7 p.m. and 7 a.m.
Having a firm understanding of modern science's approach to sleep,
as well as the Ayurvedic approach, will give you a comprehensive
understanding of how to prevent and overcome sleep ailments and
chronic tiredness.

"The alarm clock is ruining my life," my patient Calvin said in
all seriousness. "I travel constantly because of my work through two
different time zones and I have to meet my customers on time." He
called me a few days earlier introducing himself as a sales executive
with a sleep disorder. Having an older sister who had some addictive

issues with sleep medication, he was seeking a natural alternative.

I had never had anyone make such a criminal accusation of an alarm clock. I let him plead his case, "I sleep lightly all the time, but what happens is I wake up around five o'clock in the morning and I feel fine," continued Calvin. "But even though I am wide awake, I think I need more rest. Just as soon as I lie back down and fall asleep, the alarm goes off. I hit the snooze button and roll over."

"When the alarm buzzes again, it really is time for me to get up and then I feel terrible. Twenty or 30 minutes earlier I was bright-eyed and ready to go. But after hitting the snooze button (sometimes 2-3 times), everything seems to get worse."

Calvin's problem was easy to explain and he was shocked when he heard the simple truth. Like almost everyone who comes to my door, he had no knowledge of the modern understanding or the Ayurvedic understanding, of the anatomy of sleep. Once he gained a foundation of understanding, he could easily adjust his sleeping style to provide maximal rest and an optimal attitude come morning.

Understanding your sleep cycle reveals newfound freedoms that are not commonly known today. The power of this knowledge will diminish or prevent the stranglehold of dullness and fatigue. Tiredness can be so overpowering that it can drag you into unconsciousness, even while driving your car. Gaining mastery over sleep will eliminate such helplessness and will further improve your waking state the following morning. Feeling helpless to the moods and manner of how you fall asleep will also limit your options of how you will feel as you wake.

When you understand exactly what happens during sleep, then you will be able to understand why the alarm clock is a bad idea. You

> *Understanding your sleep cycle reveals newfound freedoms that are not commonly known today.*

will also come to understand why a healthy human being only needs about three hours and fifteen minutes of deep sleep and rest. Yes, you read that correctly.

When you fall asleep, you enter stage 1 of sleep where you spend 1-5 minutes gently relaxing. As you fall deeper asleep, you enter stage 2 and typically remain there for 40-50 minutes. Falling deeper into a resting state, stage 3 brings deep muscular relaxation and rest, lasting 7-15 minutes. Finally, stage 4 brings the deepest amount of rest and lasts about 12 minutes. From stage 4 you then proceed back to stage 3, then to stage 2, and then to REM (rapid eye movement sleep) which lasts about 10-30 minutes and is associated with dreaming. REM sleep, however, is not associated with muscle relaxation or rest. Then this 90-120 minute cycle repeats 2-5 times each night, culminating with a few shorter cycles which alternate between REM sleep and the second stage of sleep.

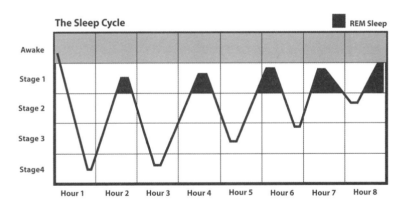

The most important characteristics of the sleep cycle are the stage 3 and stage 4 sleep periods. These are the times when you get the deepest, most restful sleep. Therefore, you really only need those two stages to feel rested; the other stages do not yield rest. The reason so many people sleep for 8 hours and wake up feeling exhausted is because they spend most of their night in sleep stages 1, 2 and REM.

However, the rest you get in stages 3 and 4 is the key to sleeping efficiently.

Furthermore, you can now be able to understand why my patient Calvin was having so much trouble with his alarm clock. When Calvin woke up at 5 a.m. feeling rested and ready to go, he was probably rising from either stage 1 or REM sleep – thus he was alert and fully awake. However, when he awoke after setting his alarm clock for an additional 30 minutes of sleep, he was then entering the deeper realms of the sleep (stage 3 or 4). Jolting up from the experience of deep sleep made him feel dull, groggy and irritated. His only error

---

Checklist for a Restless Night:
- Eating after 7:00 p.m.
- Consuming caffeine after 6:00 p.m.
- Going to sleep after 10:00 p.m.
- Exercising vigorously after 8:00 p.m.
- Watching disturbing television or movies in the hour before you go to bed.
- Listening to disquieting music in the hour before you go to bed.
- Eating spicy foods at your evening meal.
- Handling business or financial concerns the hour before you go to bed.
- Exercising (to the point of increasing your heart rate) less than four times per week.
- Allowing yourself to argue or fight with other members of the household in the hour before you go to bed.
- Drinking coffee throughout the day.
- Drinking caffeinated sodas throughout the day.

was his desire to gain 30 more minutes of sleep. When I explained the sleep cycle to Calvin, he immediately realized the importance of getting up when he felt rested and not setting the alarm.

When you realize that those 20 or 30 minutes of sleep may not offer much rest, and may also ruin your morning, it becomes much easier to get out of bed right away. Furthermore, if you wake up and feel you need more sleep, ideally, you should rest for another 90 minutes to complete another sleep cycle. Since this ideal option is rarely possible, yoga nidra offers you a wonderful solution.

Ayurvedic Sleeping – Yoga Nidra

Yoga science offers you the solutions to help you master the sleep cycle – this knowledge and this ability puts you in a rare class. The great majority of people sleep as documented by the accepted stages of sleep and the sleep cycle. This means you go from the waking state and gradually descend through four stages of sleep, landing at level 4, the home of deep sleep. It is only in stages 3 and 4 that you are truly gaining rest. However, most people do not stay in these two stages very long. Instead, shortly after reaching the state of deep sleep, you start to drift upward into the second and REM stages of sleep where dreams dominate. Thus, the goal is to maximize your time in stage 3 and particularly in stage 4, so that you can gain deep rest in a shorter period of time.

The Mandukya Upanishad is an ancient text that explores the four states of consciousness. These four basic states of consciousness are waking, dreaming, sleeping, and turiya, which is a comprehensive state beyond the others. Yoga science teaches you how to voluntarily and

> *Yoga science offers you the solutions to help you master the sleep cycle.*

freely travel between the first three states of consciousness, gaining mastery over the sleep cycles. This technique is called *yoga nidra*, or yogic sleep.

Yoga nidra offers you the unique opportunity to observe yourself interfacing with three different levels of consciousness. According to Swami Rama, yoga nidra is a state of conscious sleep. Karen and I sought to learn yoga nidra with the goal of reducing our sleep, sharpening our minds and deepening our understanding of ourselves. We knew that our identity and self-worth was too deeply entrenched in external worldly values – one bad day at the office made life at home difficult that night. We wanted to be able to rest more deeply and understand ourselves at a deeper level. Yoga nidra was the solution for us.

After several months of following Swami Rama's guidelines for yoga nidra, I wanted to test my progress in a lab. I placed three temperature diodes attached to a biofeedback machine on my forehead, throat and the center of my chest. These three locations are the physiological homes to the three common states of consciousness: waking (forehead), dreaming (throat), and sleeping (heart/center of chest). By placing your awareness at one of these three locations, you can access that state of experience. For example, in the dreaming state, your subtle awareness is unconsciously focused at the throat center. By consciously bringing your awareness to your throat with proper instruction, you will eventually be able to consciously enter the world of dreams. Many yoga texts talk about how the temperature of these three centers is influenced by the mind. When you focus your awareness on one of the three locations, then it is said that the temperature will increase at that specific location as well. Thus, it was logical that the temperature sensors would verify the focus of my concentration. Hooked up to the lab's computer, I was ready to test my concentration and verify this ancient technique.

I completed the prerequisite exercises in the lab and then began the yoga nidra practice. The biofeedback therapist gave me verbal instructions throughout the experiment and made a written record of my body's state as the computer documented the changes in my body temperature. I was asked to enter and quickly leave the throat and heart center areas. If I stayed too long at the throat center, I could get caught by a dream sequence and forget my experiment. Likewise, if I lingered at the heart center I could remain in deep sleep. As a scientist, I needed to stay sharp and actively control the focus of my mind.

The experiment lasted less than 30 minutes as we tested several rounds of concentration. The computer printouts of my body temperatures and the observations of the therapist were quite conclusive. My body temperature did change at the area of my body where my concentration was focused. At whatever site I held my attention, the temperature increased while at the other two sites the temperature simultaneously decreased. Even though my body snored when I went into deep sleep at the heart center, I felt completely conscious and was able to follow the technician's verbal instructions. This simple experiment fueled my interest in yoga nidra.

Insight through Sleep

Gaining insight and wisdom through sleep is not a concept that is limited to the tradition of yoga and the technique of yoga nidra. The famous surrealist painter Salvador Dali is reported to have taken a strange type of nap. He would place a metal pan next to a chair and then go to sleep sitting in the chair with a spoon in his hand held over the pan. As soon as he lost consciousness -- and therefore muscle control -- he would drop the spoon. The sound of the spoon clattering on the pan would awaken him. In this brief nap he claimed to find inspiration for his paintings. Thomas Edison used a remarkably similar technique to gain insights for his inventions. He would go to sleep in a chair with ball bearings in his hands. Just like Dali, he would drop them when he lost consciousness and awake inspired and ready to work.

My further reading about yoga nidra mentioned a fourth state of consciousness, called *turiya* that can be experienced through practice. This is the fully conscious state that is not lost even in the midst of deep sleep. Turiya is beyond waking, dreaming and sleeping. In turiya, you have the ability to observe yourself in deep sleep, yet you can also gain great insights and knowledge. Thus, afterwards you feel rested and may have gained newfound insights.

While yoga nidra will provide you with deep rest and rejuvenation, the ultimate goal of this practice is much more profound. Yoga nidra is "used to develop wisdom that cannot be developed otherwise... it will help you solve problems and give you solutions..." writes Swami Rama.[24] This is the power and insight that yoga nidra offers you.

> *You can learn how to achieve deep rest in a short period of time when you learn yoga nidra.*

AN INTRODUCTION TO YOGA NIDRA

You can learn how to achieve deep rest in a short period of time when you learn yoga nidra. If you spend 10-15 minutes a day practicing the inner methods of yoga nidra, you will not only feel more rested and therefore need less sleep, but you will also soon come to know yourself in a very expansive and inspiring manner.

The first prerequisite to yoga nidra is a moderate level of experience with diaphragmatic breathing, alternate nostril breathing and the 61-Point Relaxation exercise. These techniques will improve your health and increase your emotional stability. Furthermore, the sleepiness, commonly felt when learning 61 points, can be overcome through dietary modifications and repetition of the relaxation exercise. When you find it easy to breath diaphragmatically and can travel through all

61 points without falling asleep, then you are ready to learn 'Advanced Relaxation.' When you have a good understanding of these practices, you are ready to begin learning the initial stages of yoga nidra.

Yoga nidra is a multi-layered practice where you graduate to deeper and deeper levels of experience and understanding. In the beginning, you may notice that yoga nidra offers you a way to gain deep rest in a short period of time. Later you may discover that this technique will greatly benefit your insightfulness and your mental acuity. In this book, I can only provide you with a simple and effective methodology for you to begin the practice of yoga nidra. A teacher is required for the more advanced levels of this practice.

YOGA NIDRA PRACTICUM — THE FIRST STEP

After having completed the 61-Point Relaxation and Advanced Relaxation, the first step in the practice of yoga nidra begins with finding a consistent time when you are not overly tired or exhausted. If you are sleepy, you will not be able to maintain control over your states of consciousness and will easily slip into the dream world or into the typical stages of sleep.

This exercise should be done in the corpse pose* (shivasana) in a dark room, preferably before sunrise or at sunset. A small pillow should be placed under your head for comfort. You should also not have indigestion or physical discomfort when you practice yoga nidra. Do not practice this first stage of yoga nidra for more than ten minutes because you are likely to fall asleep rather than gain deep rest.

Begin by lying down in an area where phones, computers, or family members will not disturb you. While it is best to practice yoga nidra before sunrise or at sunset, choose any time that is practical for you. It is most important to continue the practice regularly at the same time of day and that your lifestyle remains consistent during the

* The corpse pose is illustrated in Chapter 5.

weeks or months that you have dedicated to learning this wonderful practice.

In the *waking state*, your awareness is focused between the two eyebrows. Close your eyes and bring your awareness to this point and take three slow diaphragmatic breaths. Next, move your attention to the throat center -- the home of dreams. Slowly and gently take 10-20 breaths while keeping your awareness at the hollow of your throat. Every breath should be simple, serene and diaphragmatic. Do not linger at your throat center or you will easily slip into the dream world.

Next, bring your attention to your heart center, located in the center of your chest not at your physical heart. Breathe here for the remainder of this practice. The heart center is the main focal point for yoga nidra. You may begin to fall asleep, but try to maintain consciousness as your breath becomes very fine. After about 10 minutes of practicing yoga nidra, start to bring your attention systematically outward. This exercise gives you the rare opportunity to consciously observe the subtle correlation between the focus of your attention and the states of consciousness.

As you gain some experience with this first level of yoga nidra, you will feel greatly re-energized after only a few minutes of this practice. When you want to explore the deeper dimensions of yoga nidra, find an experienced teacher who can guide you. Combining expert guidance, personal experience and the insights from valid texts will help you come to know about turiya and the amazing possibilities this practice can bring you.

> *Your final meal of the day strongly influences the quality of your sleep.*

SLEEP, REST, AND BE HAPPY

Sometimes understanding the sleep cycle and yoga nidra is not enough to free you from the bondage of sleep. There are eight factors that have a tremendous impact on the restfulness of your sleep. To gain deeper rest, you may need to look at these eight factors: your diet, your mind, your breath, your bedtime, your bed itself, your daytime rest, your personal sleep cycle and your waking time.

The first and most important factor for deep sleep and rest is your diet. The last four hours before bedtime are critical. In healthy adults over 25 years of age, solid foods should be avoided for approximately 3-4 hours before bedtime so that your sleep is not merely dictated by the nature of the foods you just ate. When your stomach is busy digesting foods at bedtime, then your mental function is distracted. Thus, when you do not eat solid foods for at least three hours before bedtime, then your mental fire will burn bright as you actively initiate the stages of sleep.

Furthermore, your final meal of the day strongly influences the quality of your sleep. When the last meal of the day is light, fresh and warm, your sleep will be more pleasant and restful. If your final meal of the day is spicy, oily, and lifeless (such as leftovers from previous meals or meat), then your sleep will more likely be agitated, dull, and less restful. Therefore, pay special attention to the final meal of the day.

A wonderful home remedy for insomnia is boiled milk before bedtime. Eight ounces of boiled milk with a teaspoon of sugar can be taken at bedtime and will ensure a more peaceful transition to deep sleep. The carbohydrates in the milk will encourage the release of seratonin and increased absorption of tryptophan. Seratonin is the neurotransmitter of happiness to help you sleep, and tryptophan is the amino acid that is a major building-block in the production of seratonin. Consider having a small glass of hot milk at bedtime to aid in the restfulness of your sleep.

The second most important factor for good sleep is your mind. A regular practice of meditation before bedtime will calm and cleanse the mind. It is also very important to monitor the stream of information being absorbed by your mind in the final hours before bedtime. Some of my patients had the habit of watching the news just before bedtime. They often complained of bad dreams that involved serious accidents and other types of frightening incidents. The violent and sad stories they saw on the television were actually ruining the quality of their sleep. Once they stopped watching the news before bed, their disturbing dreams ceased.

Another group of my patients suffered because their mind kept replaying the events of their day while they were lying in bed. They had a hard time getting rest because their mind was so busy running through everything that they needed to remember and complete the next day. My simple suggestion of taking ten minutes to write a list of things that they needed to do the following day helped them achieve better sleep and rest. You, too, can make a list of the urgent things that you need to remember and keep it by your bedside so that your mind is free to rest.

The third most important factor of good sleep is your breath. It is important to always breathe through your nose throughout your day. Nasal breathing helps your mental acuity and steadiness. If you are able to take the time for breathing exercises during the day, you will have much better sleep at night. The yogic texts claim that one minute of proper breathing will restore 60 minutes of vitality (pranic pressure) to your mind and body. Spending 12 minutes on focused breathing twice daily will provide you with the rejuvenative 24 minutes needed to re-vitalize yourself from the last 24 hours of your day. I ask my patients who have insomnia or other sleep disorders to learn alternate nostril breathing and practice it during those 12 minutes.

Going to bed on time is essential and is the fourth important factor for good, restful sleep. When you stay up past 10 p.m., it becomes easier to stay awake long after midnight. This is because the fire of metabolism peaks between 10 p.m. and 2 a.m. Thus, you will have a greater ability to control your sleep and get deeper amounts of rest if you are sound asleep before 10 p.m. Also, by going to bed a little earlier you will not be so exhausted at bedtime.

Your bed is also very important in your sleep habits – your bed is the fifth factor for good sleep. If your bed is overly comfortable, it can be very difficult to get out of bed in the morning. Likewise, an uncomfortable bed can make it very difficult to gain any rest. Therefore, it is important to have a bed that provides support, yet does not engulf you with too much comfort.

If it is possible, the bed can become your exclusive retreat for sleep and rest. Reading, knitting, television viewing and work activities are not bedroom activities. Keep the bed as a sanctuary for rest and relationships. It trains your mind to immediately calm down and begin to rest when you go to bed. I urge my patients with insomnia to use their bed only for sleeping.

> *When you wake up feeling refreshed and ready to go, it is important to get out of bed immediately.*

The sixth factor for good sleep is taking 10-15 minutes to rest in the afternoon. A "power nap" can help you get your edge back when done properly. As you spend more time in the deeper stages of sleep, you will naturally need less time in bed. Taking a 10- to 15-minute rest in the afternoon can further advance your ability to reduce your sleep. It is incredible how this short period of rest can help you make it through the remainder of your day with vigor and vitality. I have included the entire technique for this power nap earlier in this chapter.

The seventh factor for good sleep is to remember the difference between sleep and rest. Most people spend their sleep in stages 1 and 2 and in REM sleep. You can maximize your rest when you train your mind to go into stages 3 and 4. You can learn to rest when you practice yoga nidra and consciously control your states of sleep.

The eighth factor for good sleep is getting up on time. When you do not get out of bed on time, then your next night of sleep may also suffer. Therefore, when you wake up feeling refreshed and ready to go, it is important to get out of bed immediately. When you go to bed at 10 p.m. it becomes easier to awake by 5 a.m. It is also helpful to immediately have some water when you wake. This will make you less likely to go back to sleep.

When you follow these eight factors for deeper, more restful sleep, you will begin to have the ability to control your sleep cycle. You will need less sleep, wake up more refreshed, and feel happier throughout your day. No longer will you be enslaved by your sleep cycle. For most people, it is possible to get the equivalent of eight hours of sleep in only 4-6 hours. Therefore, follow these eight factors for good sleep, practice yoga nidra, and you will gain freedom from the bondage of sleep.

Checklist for More Restful Sleep

- A fresh, calming diet.
- Meditation before bedtime to calm and cleanse your mind.
- Take the time for breathing exercises during the day.
- Go to bed on time every night.
- Have a bed that provides support, yet does not engulf you with too much comfort.
- Take 10-15 minutes to rest in the afternoon.
- Review and remember the difference between sleep and rest.
- Get up on time.

CHAPTER SUMMARY

- *Sleep doesn't always provide good rest. It is quite possible to sleep 8 hours and still be tired if the sleep was of poor quality. Therefore, it is important to learn to sleep properly.*

- *What you eat, watch, listen to, think about and do in the hours before sleeping will affect the quality of your sleep dramatically.*

- *Through the science of yoga and the practice of yoga nidra it is possible to gain deep rest in a short period of time.*

ACTION ITEMS

- *Take note of your behaviors in the four or five hours before sleeping, and use the information presented in this chapter, along with the "checklist for a restless night" to determine which of those behaviors are helpful and which are not helpful.*

- *Begin either the prerequisite practices for yoga nidra or the actual practice of yoga nidra as described in this chapter.*

- *Experiment with not using an alarm clock. Instead, wake up immediately in the morning as soon as you feel rested and awake for the first time.*

Chapter

Creating More Space for Happiness

I was short on time, my patient schedule was over-booked, and Karen said I was wound tighter than a drum. I was about to have a very bad day. And it was bad only because I feared having an extreme shortage of time and space to fulfill all my duties. In those days I would become tense, irritable and hopeless in the face of an extremely busy day.

If I had only known many years ago that those tense moments were optional and changeable. I had no idea then how easy it is to illuminate and expand "crunch time" at the office into a field of time and space that comfortably seats every obligation.

I was not a chemistry or physics major in college, but I knew that there were solid particles smaller than the microscope could see. In the atom these tiny pieces, called electrons, whirl around the nucleus of the atom. But what caught my attention were my professor's comments that there was more space than there was solid matter. Everything solid was floating in a vast ocean of space.

The old science fiction television show "Star Trek" declared that space was "the final frontier." And many years later a yoga class proved this to be true in ways beyond my wildest imagination. In theory and in practices that can be learned, it was the science of pranayama that helped me find more space in my day.

Prana is a Sanskrit term for the first unit of energy. It is not physical, but gives life and animation to matter. When your prana is depleted, you will experience a sense of weakness and lethargy. For example, flu-like symptoms of weakness can appear in even the strongest athlete, completely overpowering the muscular strength in their heart and throughout their body. The body habitus of an athlete is no match for a lack of prana.

> *Increasing pranic pressure within you can repel stress and disease.*

Pranayama is the science of learning how to control, expand and channel prana for healing and self-transformation. When you feel depleted of enthusiasm and lack the motivation to act, yoga science would state that the pranic pressure of your body has diminished. Increasing the amount of active prana within you will also increase the amount of space in which you exist. In practical terms, a muscle spasm is skeletal tissue that is lacking space. Feeling hopeless due to a lack of options is cured by increasing your field (space) of options. Increasing pranic pressure within you can repel stress and disease. In an expanded state of mind, you are the ruling monarch of your life. Nothing can enter your space without your permission. The power and potency of prana will return your vigor and charm.

"Stretch beyond your limitations! Expand your realm of possibility. Increase your personal power!" the seminar leaders would demand. It was the 1980s and, like many of our colleagues, my wife and I enrolled ourselves in various motivational seminars. It was an era focused on the conquest of the self. What "self" actually meant varied from seminar teacher to seminar teacher. And that was ironic because, beneath the guise of "motivation," a sense of self is precisely what the attendees of these seminars were seeking. Karen and I were seeking it, too. But, in truth, we did not find it there.

The seminars inspired us to keep searching – and search we did. And as it often happens, the answer was right there in our own backyard. We were at an evening lecture in Wisconsin featuring a talk by Panditji. The moment he said, "By expanding the breath, you expand your concept of yourself." Karen and I looked at each other and grinned. He had our full attention.

"The physical body floats in a sea of primordial energy called prana," he continued. "When the physical body and the mental awareness contract, causing pain, fatigue or anguish, the unceasing bath of prana is ready to lift you up and nourish you. But like any sponge tightly held, when the death grip of fear and stress squeeze you, there is no room for

> *Hatha yoga and pranayama can expand your capacity by literally helping you stretch and expand yourself.*

prana to seep in. That is when hatha yoga and pranayama can expand your capacity by literally helping you stretch and expand yourself." Panditji continued to discuss the concept of *pranayama*. This Sanskrit word means "the control or expansion of prana."

At first, pranayama is introduced through breathing exercises that promote relaxation and a gentle lengthening of the breath. Panditji taught us several techniques for expanding our breath and our self-concept with very simple breathing exercises. As I started to practice his teachings, I realized that I was learning how to create more space in my day. Like everyone else, each year of my life was consistently becoming more hectic and hurried. These exercises were changing all of this.

The more I practiced, the more spacious my day felt and the more inspired I became about the possibilities. After several years, I felt I had finally perfected the most basic aspects of these practices – and so powerful are these basics that I found I could offer my patients a five-minute solution for resolving feelings of being "crowded, cramped, rushed and depleted." Eager to test my theories and solutions, I entered my waiting room filled with a sense of possibility.

I walked into the waiting room to find a nicely dressed pregnant woman with a face full of agony. It was obvious that her baby could arrive at any moment. For years she had worked as a physical therapist and was getting ready to birth her third child. She looked extremely unhappy as we walked back to my office with one infant in a stroller and another eager to be born. As she sat down, the tears began to well up in her eyes and I moved the Kleenex box closer to her chair. "I know you are going to think this is all hormonal, but it is not," she muttered.

"I ran track in high school and college. The sound of the starting gun gave me a thrill and I loved it all. I loved the competition, the open air and the warm sun. But now I feel like a runner who has gone mad. The starting gun has been replaced with the alarm clock and I am just so…" She drifted off into tears. I waited for her to regain her composure. I kept my attention focused on her, hoping to convey my compassion and interest in her story. After a few moments she continued.

"My life is a race from the moment the alarm clock starts buzzing. I have kids to care for, a husband to get out the door and a job to go to. You always ask me to describe how I feel about my life. Over the past month the answer has been exceedingly clear. I feel rushed, crowded, cramped and depleted. The fact that this new baby is about to join us has completely broken me." She became very quiet. She looked to the carpet for solace. I waited while the conversation continued quietly in her mind. When she was done, she glanced up. It was my turn. Sara and I had a long professional relationship and I could speak honestly and directly to her.

I agreed that I didn't think it was hormonal at all. I thought her omplaints were very honest and very common. Since Sara and I had known each other for years, I pointed out how clearly I knew that she loved her children. She smiled. And I acknowledged how much she loved her husband, who was also my patient. Her eyes brightened. I also recognized that she was feeling over-obligated and stretched way beyond her capacity. Once again, she took over the conversation.

"I do love them all but I also have to work. It seems that I am so busy that I am starting to become forgetful. One of my coworkers told me that she actually forgot to pick up her child from daycare. She only has one child, but she forgot! She said she was just too busy in her mind. I do not want that to happen to me."

Sara went on to explain, "I came to see you because I feel that my love and energy are at an all-time low." There were no tears now, just honesty. She was intelligent, desperate and entering the zone of self-condemnation simply because she was so disappointed in her ability to respond to the life that she was living. She thought she should know how to handle every situation and when she didn't and couldn't, guilt and embarrassment overcame her.

My heart opened and the words flowed from my lips. "You definitely need more space in your day. If you learn how to have more space in your day, it will feel like you have more time. *But you don't need more time, you need more space.* And creating more space is really quite easy.

"First, observe the flow of your breath right now. Gently sit still and close your eyes and observe your breathing pattern. Let your mind travel in and out of your nose with the air you are breathing. Just observe this for several breaths." She closed her eyes and sat quietly. A few moments later her eyes opened, signaling that her observations were complete.

"Lengthen your breath by just a few seconds on both inhalation and exhalation," I told her. Her eyes closed as she followed my instructions. I watched as her body settled more deeply into the chair. For the next several minutes she continued to make more space in her breath. The glow from her face and the change of her posture displayed the benefits of her lengthened breath. As she continued to gain more space in her breath, I knew that her mental clarity could further improve with a simple memory exercise that Swami Rama had been teaching for years.

Today I use the analogy of the computer's hard drive as a way to explain Swami Rama's memory technique. Our mind and a computer's hard drive both receive information to store that later can be purged and erased. Imagine the memory banks of a computer's hard drive to be like a room full of shelves. Placing various boxes of data on the shelves is how you store information. Initially, the shelves fill up in a systematic order. Over time, as you purge unneeded data, it leaves random open spaces on the shelves throughout the room. In computer lingo, this state of disarray is called a fragmented hard drive.

> *If you learn how to have more space in your day, it will feel like you have more time.*

Computer enthusiasts commonly run software to defragment their hard drives and put things back into order. This process eliminates the empty spaces and makes the hard drive run more efficiently. Swami Rama taught a memory practice that can defragment and organize your mind in a similar fashion. In the most simplistic terms, all memory is relational – meaning it is related or connected to something else in order to be found or accessed. This practice is a counting exercise that will re-establish orderliness in both an energetic and neurological manner.

"Now let's re-organize your brain," I said with a broad smile. "Bring your awareness to the point between your two eyebrows. Let your awareness hover in that area as we begin the counting exercise to improve your memory.

"As you continue to breathe through your nose in a smooth and slow manner, start to count from zero to 25 and then from 25 back to zero without a pause. Count silently to yourself, maintaining your awareness at the point between the two eyebrows. Your goal is to count this way without any pause or hesitation." Quite pleased with her accomplishment, she opened her eyes.

I explained to her that the counting would increase by units of 50 until she was able to count to 100 and back again without error or hesitation. I playfully demonstrated that this was not to be an aerobic exercise and thus she should try to avoid bouncing her head or contorting her body as each number was counted. Like all internal practices, this exercise is best accomplished while seated with the head, neck and trunk in straight alignment. The body should remain calm and still.

This practice begins with a count of 50 and is gradually increased by 50. Increasing the count is only done after perfection is achieved and maintained for several days. This perfection implies that you are able to count accurately, rhythmically and consistently for several days or more before increasing the practice. Your counting speed will dramatically increase over time. The final goal of this practice is to count to 1,000 and back perfectly. (I have wondered if the goal of a 1,000 has a correlation to the fact that every single neuron in the brain is potentially connected to 1,000 other neurons.) My experience with others and myself has shown that counting to 1,000 and back once a day for 11 days in a row yields dramatic benefits of mental clarity and memory recall. With regular practice, anyone can reach the goal of 1,000 within five or six weeks.

To increase her confidence, we counted again, this time reaching to 50 and back. She was pleased with her progress.

A few months after her child was born, she found the time to return to my office and report her progress. Upon this occasion when I entered the waiting room to greet her, it was obvious that she had found her joy and vigor again. I introduced myself to the newborn baby as we strolled back to my office.

"I think every woman should be taught that counting exercise, especially when pregnant!" she exclaimed. "In my last few days of pregnancy when I was bored and uncomfortable, your counting exercise was a great way to pass the time." I smiled at the thought of this new opportunity for teaching the memory exercise. She continued to tell me how her hurriedness and over-crowdedness seemed less prominent as she continued to expand the length of her breath. Breathing exercises were noticeably easier for her to perform after her new daughter had been born. Even though her duties had greatly increased by caring for her newborn, her capacity to do it all was back. And along with it, her joy was back, too.

She talked at length about her improved memory and the benefits of practicing her breathing. Breath work was not new to her, for she was an avid student of hatha yoga and it was her instructor that had referred her to my clinic years ago. She was quite familiar with the 61-Point Relaxation exercise and mentioned that she practiced this exercise several times a week. I knew that her life would only continue to get busier now that she was the mother of three children all under the age of 5. Since she had a regular practice of the 61-Point Relaxation exercise, I knew that she was ready for something more. She needed something to further expand her capacity to embrace and utilize all of the daily challenges that every working parent faces.

I paused to reflect because we had been at this point together before. I could feel her intrigue. Because of her experience with hatha and breathing practices, she knew of the concept of creating space within her mind and body. The counting exercise had been a marvelous tool for Sara and now she was ready to learn the 'advanced relaxation' technique that I discussed in chapter seven.

"Advanced relaxation is a true practice of pranayama – it expands the amount of space and prana within you," I began. "As your mental awareness and breath travel together in this exercise, you will be creating more room within you. You will stretch and expand the flow of prana which will remove subtle waste and anxiety. As your pranic pressure increases, your enthusiasm and confidence will increase.

"Sara, advanced relaxation techniques can create more space for you in even your busiest day. It is important to do this accurately, so follow these instructions and contact me when you have practiced for a few weeks. It is common that people overlook a few details of this practice, so that is why we should re-visit the technique when you are ready."

Sara and I discussed the practice in regards to arranging time in her day and the importance of quietness. She decided that she would start the exercise on a weekly schedule for the next three months. Inspired to take the next step with this advanced relaxation practice, we ended our appointment.

Each week I continue to help people of all ages create more space in their life. To some it feels as if the days are longer in a manner that they feel less hurried. To others, they feel so much more productive that it seems they are stretching time – accomplishing several hours of work in less than 60 minutes.

Their feedback and enthusiasm spurred Karen and I to keep practicing these same techniques in our lives. As we continued to learn, study and practice, we also noticed that the "time continuum" was changing from a Hollywood fantasy into an experiential fascination. In the next chapter we will explore the concept of time and time management.

CHAPTER SUMMARY

- *You can't change time, but you can change your experience of time by creating more space, flexibility and vitality in your body through the practice of hatha yoga and pranayama.*

- *Controlling your breath is the quickest way to control your mind. Your breathing patterns have great influence over your experience of life.*

ACTION ITEMS

- *Set aside a practical amount of time everyday for yourself to stretch and work with your breath using the alternate nostril breathing technique, described in Chapter 7, and hatha yoga exercises from Chapter 5 of this book.*

- *Try the counting exercise explained in this chapter for 11 days.*

- *Create a practical but consistent schedule to experiment with the Advanced Relaxation exercise outlined in chapter 7.*

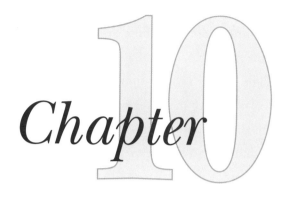

Chapter

Filling Your Day with Happiness

Hippocrates said, "Healing is a matter of time, but it is sometimes also a matter of opportunity." I agree with him. However, I feel that most of us do not take the opportunity time provides us.

One of my professors joked that the purpose of time is to prevent everything from happening at once. And yet, when I talk to my overstressed patients, it seems to them that everything *is* happening at the same time. In the pursuit of happiness, time management is absolutely essential.

Time provides structure to your life and it is the light of the sun that provides structure to time. Modern life is starting to obscure the sun and the moon from being visual frames of reference. Fewer of my patients can respond affir-

> *In the pursuit of happiness, time management is absolutely essential.*

matively to my questions, "Did you see the beautiful sunrise today? Did you notice the color of the moon last night?" The human race is starting to go inside – into condos, office buildings and massive shopping malls. The more disconnected we become from the source of the time principle - the sun - the more difficult time management will be. Many say that time is too precious to waste, yet they lack the skills needed to make the best use of it because they have lost contact with the sun and the moon. The science of Ayurveda can help you re-establish this link between your life and your time.

Ayurveda states that the first step in time management is to recognize that your emotions from yesterday are still influencing you today. If you go to bed angry or worried, you will wake up angry or worried. In this sense, sleep acts only as a slight recess from the feelings that inhabit your waking moments. Your bedtime mood will usually determine your morning experience. Freedom comes when you apply this whole new way of thinking about time to every day and, especially, every night.

Attaining your goals is much easier when you understand the secret relationship between yourself and time. For thousands of years, Ayurveda has provided a systematic way of allowing people to determine their own constitution and discover the optimal way to use every hour of the day. With just a little bit of knowledge, you can make time work for you. This ancient science is still accurate today.

THE LARGER BLOCKS OF TIME

To utilize the time principle to your advantage, you must understand what we have done to time in the past 50 years. Prior to the last half-century or so, it was common to speak about time in terms of months and years. When people thought about managing their time, they began by making New Year's resolutions. Everyone knew that when New Year's Day arrived, they could start fresh with new goals and new plans. In all cultures, humanity paused once a year to consider how they would better their life in the upcoming year.

Such seemingly long spans of time allowed us to adjust to changes in our lives and in our world. Whenever there is a rapid cascade of changes with no time for these changes to be assimilated into the human psyche, people feel rushed and disconnected.

Today, one year seems like too large a chunk of time to fathom, and yet it may take several years for the filter of time to purify that which disrupts our lives. I remember listening to Panditji counsel a couple going through huge marital strife. He said it would take three to five years for them to rebuild their trust and friendship. To me, it seemed burdensome to provide them with such a large timetable for healing. But as I watched the couple mend during that time, they told me it was actually a relief to know they could take all the time they needed to relight the flame of love that had bonded them.

While we demand instant messages and overnight shipping, the ancient sages looked at life in much larger blocks of time. They divided the human life span into four blocks of time that totaled 100 years. While such a full life is not yet common, they painted a fascinating picture of how we could spend our life in a manner conducive to self-understanding and service to all.

> *To be born
> and never uncover
> the highest joy in life
> would be a great loss.*

The first 25 years of life are devoted to learning about the world. During this time, you come to know yourself and gain enough worldly knowledge to live comfortably. The ages of 25 to 50 are devoted to the childbearing years, when you raise a family and become established in your community. This phase of life helps maintain the broader social and community foundations that allow a society to survive and thrive.

In the transition to the third phase of life, you complete all of your family obligations and begin reflecting upon the meaning and purpose of life. According to the sages, to be born and never uncover the highest joy in life would be a great loss. This third phase of life, from ages 50 to 75, is the time to uncover that joy. Life now affords you the time to further polish your self-understanding under the tutelage of mentors endowed with the wisdom of direct experience. Seeking the insights and compassion of such teachers is how this time period is spent.

The golden years, from ages 75 to 100, are the time for offering your personal insights and wisdom to your family and community. Having lived a fulfilling life endows you with the knowledge and happiness that can sustain future generations.

What would happen if you and your family started a time management plan by viewing the lives of you and your children in 25-year blocks of time?

Whether you plan your life in such huge dimensions or not, most of us unconsciously accept and commit ourselves to the first two seasons of life – the time for learning, and the time to raise a family. The later times in our maturity for reflection and conclusion are slipping from our awareness. This loss of future possibilities that can finally remove all of the angst and anxiety is a modern tragedy. Our lifespan can allow time for this personal analysis and also include the time for sharing unconditionally with everyone in our golden years. As the baby-boomers age, can we encourage them to mature their own self-understanding so that they have something of value to pass on to their children and grandchildren? In the last several decades, modern societies have focused only on providing an inheritance of wealth and property. Today, the golden nuggets that our children need are entrenched in the casings of love, wisdom and the arts. Today's generations are starving for the insights of how to be happy and healthy. Gleaning these fortunes of knowledge from their elders far exceeds the value of property and material wealth.

This is the essence of time management. Every age group needs time to receive and time to give; but more importantly, we can schedule time to understand ourselves, our relationships and the purpose of our existence.

To schedule time for such lofty and vital activities begins with maintaining a daily schedule that meets the most basic human needs. If you are hungry, overly tired or conflicted, the contemplation of higher thoughts will never dawn on your awareness. Nature provides a very simple time management program. The sages organized it so that all of us can use this program and benefit from it, even if we reside inside the largest condominiums or indoor shopping malls. This philosophy allows you to make the best use of what you already have, both your strengths and your weaknesses. Your worldly desires and activities will not deplete your inner resources because you have time for both.

When I talk to my patients seeking psychotherapy, their goals for better time management always seem to center around one of three objectives: trying to fix their past, trying to let go of their past or trying to change their desires for the future. When I talk with members of the business community, whose lives revolve around deadlines and production schedules, their time management is similar. They want to repeat or not repeat the past, depending upon its financial success. They are trying to recover from bad days in the market or they are consumed with future revenues that keep escaping their grasp. Likewise, the parents that come through my

> *The only escape from the past is to live in the present — a present that remains uncontaminated by the past.*

door want a better life for their children. Their goals, like the others, are based upon repeating what worked, avoiding what didn't work and forecasting achievements for their children that may not be realistic or beneficial.

For all of these groups of people, time management is structured around either avoidance or anticipation of a time period that has passed or does not yet exist. There is no *now* in their life. Their struggles revolved around every time period *except* the present moment.

To help them I presented a little bit of knowledge that drastically reduced their fears. The myth of holding someone else responsible for your pain guarantees failure and unlimited delays. A limited grasp of the concept of self-reliance creates these myths of blame and only leads to hatred and fear. It is this lack of inner understanding that cause these errors. Exaggerating blame into an unchangeable destiny is essentially useless in every religious, psychological and spiritual pursuit.

> *Now is always the best time to let go of the past.*

Time management gives you unlimited options and power to take control of your life and stop blaming others. I use this example with my patients: "Imagine I offended you three years ago and you did not get up and slap me. Now, it is three years later and you still hate me. You still want to slap me and, yet, now you are hearing that I have changed my life. I used to be an angry man who hurt my family, but now I realize how much I was hurting myself and others. Thus, I have changed for the better.

"Now the consequences of the past are in your hands. You have the power in this present moment to make everything better or everything worse. It completely depends upon how you react to me right now. To forgive and to forget will free us both, to attack and retaliate is to renew the cycle of hurt and blame. The only escape from the past is to live in the present – a present that remains uncontaminated by the past."

We can learn how to transform our reactions to the past and thus turn the consequences of past actions and experiences in our favor. This is what *Ralph* did in Chapter 3 as he was learning to be kind to himself. Furthermore, there is no need to delay a good thing. *Now* is *always* the best time to let go of the past. When the present moment is too thick with emotions and distractions, then the next best time to work on your tough issues is when you are in a great mood. Times when you are happy and content are powerful moments for self-transformation.

It takes effort. Trying to improve your life only when you are living in troubled times is not the best plan. When things in your life are fine, that is the time to overcome your weaknesses and work hard on freeing your mind from the time sequences of the past. *Once again, work on your tough issues when you are in a great mood.* In the Bible, Jesus says, "Are there not twelve hours in the day? A man can walk in the daytime without stumbling because he has the light of this world to see by; but if he walks at night, he stumbles, because there is no light to guide him."[25] You can achieve great success in your own self-transformation by striving to be happier and healthier in the light of alertness, restfulness and playful-

> *Work on your tough issues when you are in a great mood.*

ness. Change things for the better when it is easy and when your entire physiology is there to support you.

COMPRESSING TIME

While the sages used 25-year blocks to plan their time, we plan our time with stopwatch accuracy. Every second seems precious and programmed. We are not allowed to be 10 minutes late for work. We cannot ignore our cell phone for two minutes. Our scheduling has become microscopically precise, and we use this cultural insanity to build our reputations. We have spoiled ourselves -- and we love it.

We love to ship packages overnight and know that they are absolutely, positively guaranteed to arrive before the next business morning. I can set the cruise control on my car to maintain a steady speed and thus easily predict the time of my arrival at a seminar. Our ability to obey the schedule in our office day planners does not seem to cross over into our private life. It amazes me how we have so much trouble getting ourselves to go to bed on time and yet we wake up on time in a world where we can guarantee our client that the package will arrive before 10:30 in the morning. Our priorities are out of sequence. We have conquered time in the business and computer worlds but not in our personal lives. And really, when we lie on our deathbed, which will matter more?

We cram as many activities into our day as possible. Today's typical family includes both parents racing the clock from early morning until late at night. They have children to wake and feed, lunchboxes to fill, clothes to iron, a carpool schedule to meet – and this is just the first 90 minutes of their day. The evening hours are no different, filled with cooking, homework, laundry and dishes. This compression of time may be a collective agreement in society, but it is not without loopholes for those who seek them. It is these loopholes in the law of karma that allows us to change the outcome of our most immediate and most forgotten actions. Time management is the skill of using the clock and personal diplomacy to create options instead of obstacles.

Here is the good news: you can wake-up refreshed and energized every day. To do so, you will need to learn how to cooperate with time on a very personal level. This will help you to enjoy, not just survive, the first 90 minutes of the day, regardless of how busy they are.

COOPERATING WITH TIME

It seems easy to cooperate with gross elements of time – such as the four seasons or night and day. Following the logic of time, you plant in the spring and harvest in the fall. You hang your laundry when the sun is shining. You wake up in the morning and you go to bed at night. Without acknowledging that these actions cooperate with nature, you will miss the benefits of synchronizing your actions with the rhythms of nature. It is important to do things on time. The right action at the right time will yield a maximal result. For instance, if I go to my bank to apply for a loan at midnight, my efforts will not yield the maximal result I am seeking. There is both a science and a philosophy to learning how to time your actions to circumstances most favorable to inner and outer harmony. Learning to cooperate with the rhythm of time is learning to live a life that makes sense.

I have noticed that modern science is busy documenting when problems occur, while the ancient sciences of Ayurveda focus on the optimal times to take action. When you have knowledge of both sciences, it becomes logical to cooperate with time.

> *Learning to cooperate with the rhythm of time is learning to live a life that makes sense.*

There are reasons that science can document and verify why we are best-suited to live according to the rhythms of nature.

For example, your liver functions best between 10 p.m. and 2 a.m. to cleanse the foods in your intestines. For the liver to do its work, you should be lying down and preferably asleep. It is also helpful for no new foods to be introduced into the digestive tract for at least three hours before the cleansing time begins. Thus, it is best not to eat after 7 p.m.

If you need time for creative thoughts and inspiration, science shows that the early morning hours before and at sunrise are optimal for this activity. Likewise, if you want to exercise to lose weight, Ayurveda mentions that the morning time is best.

Here are some more instances where modern medicine has revealed the importance of time in the human body.

OPTIMAL TIMES FOR DISEASE AND THERAPIES

Asthma – Asthmatic episodes most commonly occur between 3 a.m. - 5 a.m.

Heart attacks – These attacks are 40% more likely to occur between 6 a.m. – 12 p.m.[26]

Hot flashes – Most commonly occur at night

Inflammatory diseases – Most commonly flare-up in the morning

Ulcers – Aggravated in the early hours of sleep

Melatonin – Excreted from 2 a.m. – 4 a.m.

Allergic rhinitis – Usually worse in the early morning

Chemotherapy – More effective in the afternoon[27]

Blood pressure – Highest in morning (approx 7 a.m.) and lowest at 3 a.m. [28]

RHEUMATOID ARTHRITIS AND OSTEOARTHRITIS

Rheumatoid arthritis can be distinguished from osteoarthritis by the time of day when the patient's joints are most painful. Morning stiffness is characteristic of rheumatoid arthritis, whereas symptoms in the afternoon and evening often are associated with osteoarthritis. [29]

Now, let's look at Ayurveda's approach to time management. It centers on when to optimally take various types of action. When you understand this science, you can make all of your actions more successful.

YOUR CONSTITUTION'S ROLE IN TIME MANAGEMENT— MAKING TIME WORK FOR YOU

Every hour of the day, every day of the week and every season of the year can work in your favor if you know both a little bit about yourself and a little bit about timing. Initially, Ayurveda divides your day into six separate four-hour blocks of time. Depending upon your constitution, certain activities will be more successful when performed during the proper time period.

Specific times of the day and night affect you, regardless of your constitution. Here are the times of the day that correspond to the three Ayurvedic constitutions as we discussed in Chapter 2.

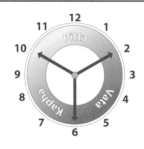

Kapha is dominant from 6 a.m. – 10 a.m.
and from 6 p.m. – 10 p.m.
Pitta is dominant from 10 a.m. – 2 p.m.
and from 10 p.m. – 2 a.m.
Vata is dominant from 2 p.m. – 6 p.m.
and from 2 a.m. – 6 a.m.

This timetable serves as an owner's manual for your mind and body. It will only take a few days to adjust your daily routine to gain optimal function and maximal happiness, putting you at the peak of your function. To have a wonderful and productive life, consider these tips in planning your day, beginning at bedtime:

1. Remember that **your day actually begins the night before.** Assuming your bedtime is 10 p.m., it is important to be cautious with your last activities of the day -- between 6 p.m. and 10 p.m. If your last waking moments are exhausting, upsetting, or irritating, you will most likely wake up exhausted, upset or irritated. Your bedtime mood determines your morning experience. Be happy.

2. When the fire of Pitta is fully awakened during its night shift (10 p.m. – 2 a.m.), this vitality is for cleansing, digesting and rejuvenation of the body. This is the time when Pitta cleanses your blood and skin of waste. However, if you are awake, the fire goes to your mind instead of cleansing your body. That is why if you stay awake past 11 p.m., it will be easy for you to stay awake until 2 a.m., which may also make you feel hungry or irritable. Thus, it is important to get into bed before Pitta wakes up (10 p.m. – 2 a.m.) at night. Sleeping from 10 p.m. until at least 4 or 5 a.m. will allow the metabolic fire of Pitta to work its wonders.

3. Waking up during Vata time (before 6 a.m.) will give you increased alertness and cheerfulness. Vata controls your nervous system and your alertness; thus, if you start your day during Vata time, you will have more energy and greater endurance throughout the day. Waking up after 6 a.m. puts you into Kapha time, when you may experience dullness, heaviness and fatigue. Stiffness, water retention and bags under the eyes are signs of imbalanced Kapha. If you rise after 6 a.m., you may wake up tired, especially if you have a Kaphic constitution.

4. The first half of the day feels more happy and hopeful because the light increases in warmth and brightness throughout the morning. The light and heat of the sun sustain not only the life on our planet but also our enthusiasm. Sunrise is inspirational; it's the reason we say "good morning." Kapha time begins at 6 a.m. and continues until 10 a.m. It is a time for you to exert your strength and demonstrate your stamina and coordination. It is a wonderful time to exercise and get things done. Be productive during the morning time of Kapha.

5. During the daytime hours of Pitta (10 a.m. – 2 p.m.) it is optimal to feed your mind the most difficult problems to be solved or the most important information to be studied. Likewise, the fire of digestion is at its peak; thus, it is often suggested that you have your heartiest, heaviest meal at noon instead of in the evening.

6. Vata time produces the greatest amount of creative energy. Schedule time for contemplation, artistic works and insight during Vata time of 2 p.m. - 6 p.m. This is also the time for fellowship and reflection. The early morning Vata time of 2 a.m. - 6 a.m. is reserved for self-reflection and fellowship with your conscience, and the afternoon period of Vata time is for creative fellowship with your friends, coworkers and family. This is when you make your lists of the next day's needs so that you do not carry them home with you or into your dreams. Brainstorming new ideas and concepts is most productive during Vata times of the day.

The Seasons

The three Ayurvedic constitutions also have their own corresponding seasons of the year. The season of each constitution is the time period that has the propensity to challenge the strength of that specific constitution. Knowing these seasons gives you an advance warning when your constitu-

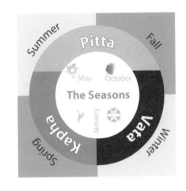

tion might be at risk if you are already facing health challenges or extraordinary stress.

For example, the cold and damp season of the year – usually the February snows through the spring rains of May – are the risky times for the health of a Kapha. An unhealthy person with a Kapha constitution will be more prone to sinus infections, bronchitis or depression during this time.

Likewise, the summer months of June through September correspond with the constitutional themes of heat and fire (Pitta). The hot temper of Pittas can be easily aroused both in the heat of competition and beneath the hot summer sun. It is important for Pittas to stay cool.

Furthermore, the Vata constitution is easily disturbed by the cold dry winds of the fall season – commonly October through January. It is easy for people with a Vata constitution to stay healthy during this Vata season by simply covering themselves from the harsh winds and being sure to stay warm.

Even a small amount of knowledge that helps you coordinate your efforts with nature's time clock can drastically reduce your ailments and stress. Becoming more aware of the fact that you live on a planet should not make you feel small and minute, but rather it should make you feel supported and connected to a much larger system of humanity and happiness. All of us want to be distinguished and behave in a polished and refined manner. Time management will give you access to these aspects of your personality. Gradually, you will be able to start your day on time and end your day on time. You will feel the formative importance of the first 25 years of your children's life and simultaneously honor the importance of bringing your commercial life to its culmination near your 50th year of life. The value of time well spent brings immeasurable good now and for years to come.

I hope the previous pages will help you find greater clarity and purpose in how you conduct your years, days and weeks throughout your life. The urge to accomplish more every day continues to grow. In our rush to achieve, the skillfulness and integrity of our actions can easily be ignored. Honoring time means to recognize the influences and relationships of past, present and future actions. The moment you see this connection is the moment you realize that the skillfulness of your next action may lead you closer to attaining your goals – both personal goals and career goals.

You realize the importance of working hard on the most difficult topics and issues when you are in the most inspired and creative mood. The time to work hard is when things are fine and flowing. It is important to realize how powerfully your skillful actions today influence your possibilities for tomorrow. When your mind and body perform in coordination with the forces of nature, then you have greatly enhanced your probability for success.

The essence of time management is knowing when to act. Your timing can be based on a combination of factors that are now becoming known to you. When you are inspired, rested and nourished … take action.

Chapter Summary

· *You can change the influence of your past experiences by changing your perception of the past.*

· *There are natural rhythms to time and to our experience of life. If you understand and cooperate with these rhythms, your life will flow more smoothly and you will struggle less.*

· *Thinking about and planning your life in 25 year blocks of time will help you lead a life that will be fulfilling to you and allow you to work toward uncovering the highest joy in life. At the same time this attitude contributes toward the maintenance of a stable and productive society.*

Action Items

· *Write down the things from your past which you are still actively involved in trying to change or simply never let go of. Consider the freedom that you would gain by letting go of these experiences.*

· *Regardless of your actual age, decide which of the four phases of life discussed in this chapter you are in right now. Then contemplate how you would like your life to be in the remaining phases and plan out what you need to do to make those visions a reality.*

· *Review the times of the day when each Ayurvedic constitution is dominant and which activities are most favorable during these times. Take note of how much of your life fits into this pattern and how much is in conflict with it. Experiment with changing those conflicting activities and notice the results.*

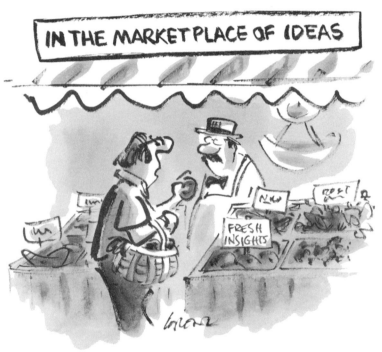

"Just how fresh are these insights?"

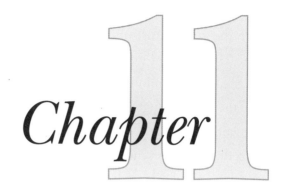

Chapter 11

A Life of Balance and Harmony
Contemplation and Your Inner World

Contemplation and meditation are complementary practices. Without contemplation, meditation becomes a mental exercise and without meditation, contemplation becomes mere imagination. With the help of contemplation, a person comprehends reality intellectually and with the help of meditation, he experiences the reality within. Through contemplation, one comes to know. Through meditation, one comes to realize. Contemplation is a prerequisite for meditation, for unless one knows intellectually that there are higher levels of reality beyond mundane phenomena, he will not begin his quest to experience those levels of reality.

The proper method for practicing contemplation and meditation is not described clearly in the texts of Vedanta philosophy; rather it is directly taught by the teacher to the student.[30]

-- Pandit Rajmani Tigunait, PhD.,

I have spent years trying to live a balanced, harmonious life. However, the fickle nature of my mind continued to spoil my progress. Having spent many years doing mantra meditation, I was disappointed that my mind still roamed the galaxy while I was trying to meditate. I was taught that contemplation and meditation are complementary practices. When contemplation and determination work together, they prevent the subconscious mind from controlling the conscious mind. I needed to constantly remind myself that the power of strong determination is greater than the urges of the subconscious mind. This seemingly simple statement became material for years of reflection.

> *The power of strong determination is greater than the urges of the subconscious mind.*

When I see people walking down the street, completely withdrawn into their internal world, I study their facial expressions. It is fascinating to watch their smiles or grimaces reflect the joyful or troubling content of their internal dialogues. We all talk to ourselves. Contemplation is the art of skillfully guiding that conversation. Such a skill eluded me due to a lack of understanding and a lack of practice.

For years I was unknowingly expanding the content of my conscious and subconscious mind with impulsive and mundane memories. When you fill the internal storage units of your mind, fill them with gold, not garbage.

According to the sages, there was a time when the size of the subconscious mind was very small and we had easier conscious access to many things. Today we use a very small part of our brain consciously. Unfortunately, we are no longer taught or warned about the repercussions of the distractions that arise from constantly filling our mind with sensory input that we will later see as a worthless waste.

I had kept myself busy making my mind more and more congested. I had prided myself on staying up on the news and being an informed person. I memorized popular songs, clever jokes and dialogues from my favorite television shows. I was innocently and needlessly expanding my chitta (the warehouse of the mind) – resulting in a mind jumbled with ideas and notions, most of which were not mine. Yoga science says that "chitta" houses the conscious and subconscious mind and the entire mind field for which we may not have a name. I was expanding my mind with the wrong stuff. Constructive contemplation would be like spring cleaning. I would get rid of the old in order to create clean, bright spaces of calm inside.

Merging my tiny wakeful mind with the consciousness of my very being should be simple. It is just me joining up with me. I tried to do it. My mind did stay quiet for a little while, but nothing constructive happened. Soon distractions from within me took over.

There is tremendous power in the contents of your chitta and some of those contents are commonly in opposition to your higher goals. If you have seen a beer advertisement 40,000 times in your lifetime, that advertisement has a lot of power. If your scripture says something bad about beer, you think, "So what?" You read your scriptures a couple of times a year and you have seen beer advertisements 40,000 times. The scriptures are overpowered and overrun with the landslide of media marketing playing in your mind.

> *We all talk to ourselves and contemplation is the art of skillfully guiding the conversation.*

"How weak is the knowledge we gain from the conscious mind? Very weak! And see how powerful the impressions are in the subconscious mind – as seen in gambling addiction, alcoholism, etc." It was Panditji again. "When you learn to see most news and information as global and technical gossip, then you start minding your own business."

I had to transform my worldview. Panditji continued, "Keep what you want to accomplish visible right in front of your eyes all the time. Keeping your higher purpose and goal in life always in front of you will make it easy for you to focus on your main primary business. Thus, you will not get scattered.

"There is a lot of pressure on us to run around and become scattered. Practice means making an effort to stay where you are. Stay focused. Stay in touch with your conscience and keep your conscience focused on your highest goals. Set up your daily and yearly priorities based on what you know that you must achieve in this life. Decide how much time you want to spend on less important things."

It became my main priority. Every morning while the world was still asleep, I would descend to the living room to sit and contemplate. "Do not get distracted by things that are not your priority," I would chant to myself over and over. I always make time to sit, eat, breathe, walk, study, do my practice and do my job.

> *When your possessions become a burden, you must discard them to go forward.*

Good focus from strong determination keeps you from getting distracted. The distinction between needs and desire is another important discovery. Most people will aimlessly run after the objects of their desire. These charms and temptations only have power over you when you do not know your purpose in life. This is why self-reflection, self-study and contemplation are so important.

Once you understand the nature of the world and the objects of the world, then you will know how to live in the world. When your possessions become a burden, you must discard them to go forward. I was ready and willing to let go of anything.

I learned early in my childhood about the power of contemplation, simply through observation. My father would spend hours in his study, reading and reflecting on the writings of Socrates, Aristotle, Plato, Shakespeare and Tolstoy. As a young boy, I only knew this to be quiet time, but somehow I knew it was also important.

I never confronted my father with my observations until one day when my older sister and I realized that our father was escaping from church, on a regular basis, before the sermon even began. One Sunday, with my sister away, I spied his escape and followed him. I got caught.

Father was not mad, but rather instructional and direct as he espoused his opinion of church-going. He sat me down on the front steps of the church and we had a father-son heart-to-heart.

> *If you see something you admire in God's personality or actions, then imitate that, embrace that.*

"If I had my way, I would focus on community service more than singing praises," he began. "Does God really need your praise? Instead, if you see something you admire in God's personality or actions, then imitate that, embrace that. You have to do the work. Do not beg him to help you, you must help yourself. I do not offer God my weaknesses, instead I offer him my strengths and talents. Without taking action and personal responsibility, worshipping alone could make you weak and dependent. God would not like that. God needs your help and the best form of help is to imitate his behaviors, to be His servant by doing His work. When you are doing His work, then you are doing the same work that He does – you inspire, teach, heal and forgive."

"If you feel that God is kind, then try to be nicer to your sister. Be kind, if that is what you find attractive in God. If you feel that God is wise, then try to do better in school. Study hard instead of arguing with your mom at homework time. If you believe God is forgiving, then forgive others and forgive yourself. To do this will take a lifetime of training, trials and errors. But you can do it and then you truly are helping God.

"Blair, I am a businessman, and though I once wanted to be a minister, I became a school teacher and eventually went into business. As a businessman, I do my very best to inspire, educate and help my clients and staff because that is my talent. When my own business partners cannot see what I see, it hurts me and I struggle with this. I come here to my office because I do not need to be lectured about God. My world is the world of business. I strive for excellence and to be helpful, that is how I worship God. I, too, do my best to imitate Him in the best way I can.

"This is my private request of you: please think about how you can help God. Do not worship Him. Instead, imitate Him. If you start to think this way now, then, someday, when you are grown up, you will be his finest servant."

And on that note our father-son meeting was adjourned. My head and my heart were full of wonder and respect. It would be 40 years or more before I would commit this private meeting to paper and finally understand how the power of my father's contemplations brought a life changing lesson to me at the grand old age of nine.

It is Important to Have an Effective Filter

Mary had thought a lot about change. She sincerely wanted to improve her life and conquer her chronic anxiety. She actively participated in my meditation classes and privately meditated at home. She wrote in her journal. She prayed for guidance. She became a vegetarian. She tried everything she knew to become happy – religion, self-help and traditional psychotherapy – but any improvement she saw was slight at best.

She was busy doing all the right things in all the right ways, but her efforts were mechanical in nature. She exercised, she prayed, she ate the "right" foods. But it was all a drill, it wasn't real. She was living proof of what happens when you do not combine your mind and heart in your efforts. For Mary, contemplation was the missing piece.

Every person needs time to think things through. Many important decisions - at home and at work -- need your attention regularly. When you are clear with your own values and integrity, these decisions can be made easily and quickly. Contemplation can help you follow through with your decisions by helping you obtain and maintain inner clarity. It empowers you to put your knowledge into action. When your actions are based on well-thought-out personal choices that you have made, they are an extension of your decisive determination. You become fully invested in every activity and event in your life.

Ironically, while Mary was coming to me for guidance, she became my teacher. It just so happened that I, too, was at a crossroads. I had hit a plateau in my own journey to self-understanding. She made me realize that we both were sitting back and witnessing our own efforts. Neither of us had fully committed to the changes we were seeking.

When things went wrong in my life, I habitually asked "Why?" If no one was near me, still the "why" questions would surface. Denying to myself that *I* could answer the questions, I chose to ignore them. Mary seemed to have the same habit. We were both still in the "somebody-out-there-knows-the-answer" mode – and we blamed them for not stepping up and answering our questions. Thus, she and I believed we remained innocently blameless and helpless. We were wasting huge amounts of time and energy.

Mary's story turned the lights on in my own mind. I immediately saw the flaws in her methods *and* in mine. As I made the discovery in my own life, I helped her realize that she had to change from the inside out. The change had to come from *her* decision, not from her guilt and not from others who teased her. She could no longer allow her mind to run in the same old circles. She had to guide her mind into thinking and believing in the manner that she wanted to think and believe.

She started to formulate a more lofty view of herself and her life. Through contemplation, she confronted her inner fears by asking herself some truthful questions: *Does it really matter what other people think of me? Who should be the top priority in my life? At this time, it is me. Others will come and go in my life — this has always been true — but I am my constant companion and I must answer to me. My actions and choice must first be acceptable to me.*

This simple dialogue marked the beginning of Mary's journey to true self-respect. She was starting to recognize how important she was to herself. She started making progress again by taking her insights gained through contemplation into her meditation practice. Her new perspective allowed her to let old thought patterns fall away. Furthermore, her contemplation dialogue helped her acknowledge and expand the positive glimpses of herself that she was gaining.

Her years of external strife started diminishing and her inward journey of contemplation had become fruitful. Her time spent in meditation and contemplation became alive and fascinating. She witnessed how her mind worked – what impulses commonly arose, what strengths she had, and how her "apparent weaknesses" were actually just habits. Those habits were much weaker than her new determination to live a happier and healthier life. Contemplation gave her unshakeable determination and brought immediate real change. Supported by her meditation, she started to think of herself and her world in new ways.

In tandem with Mary, I was experiencing similar benefits. In years past I had studied contemplation with little forward movement. In the Bible, St. Paul listed some positive virtues and encouraged us to "Think on these things."**[31] Great advice, but I couldn't do it. I literally did not know how. I honored the great minds of ancient times, but I could not follow their instruction. At that time I had been meditating for several years and progress was very slow. Inspired by books like *Autobiography of a Yogi* and *Living with Himalayan Masters*, I was expecting life-changing results and a little mysticism on the side. Working with Mary turned on the lights in my own study of contemplation as I realized the importance of willpower and determination.

THE ROLE OF PERCEPTION IN CONTEMPLATION

"Perception depends on the perceiver. Understand the role of your own perception and learn how to mold your own perception." It was Panditji offering me this wonderful freedom to view myself in any manner that I wanted. He taught the art of adjustment – how to transform your own worldview and how to transform the place where you live and work into an arena for personal development. Your own perspective on life, and on yourself, can powerfully sway your progress in self-transformation. Contemplation is the methodology for brightening and broadening your options and perspectives.

It is wonderful to see others in a good light and work hard to improve the world around you, but your "worldview" must include you.

** *Philippians 4:8, "Finally, brethren, whatsoever things are true, whatsoever things are honorable, whatsoever things are just, whatsoever things are pure, whatsoever things are lovely, whatsoever things are of good report; if there be any virtue, and if there be any praise, think on these things."*

If you really want to be happy, transform how you view yourself. For instance, a small group of my patients were volunteers for wonderful humanitarian projects – they built houses, served food and loved all. Whenever a great cause came along, they were the first to sign up! They were completely devoted to helping others. However, in spite of their altruism, they were not happy at their core. They had cultivated unending compassion for others, but had completely forgotten to extend that same compassion to themselves; thus they suffered from disappointment and dismay from their own errors. Contemplating on their compassion toward others could lead them to adopt a similar attitude toward themselves. It would be a simple but vital addition to their self-concept. Without including themselves in their attitude of selfless service, they may someday feel used and taken advantage of by the very humanitarian organizations they now endear.

For most of us, contemplation is a learned art; for others it is a life-long tendency. It was later in life that I came to learn and understand this skill. For more than half of my life I did not know how to think about my thinking process or myself. Contemplation was just a word, a lofty term for sophisticated minds, but not a reality for me.

> *Contemplation is not a skill limited to the spiritual seeker, rather it is an essential skill for every man, woman and child.*

Like many children, I was sent to my room when I erred to "think about what I had done wrong." While I thought I had accomplished this mission, in truth, all I had done was master the art of self-condemnation. My parents, like many, may not have fully explained the goal of my time in solitude. I was supposed to process the lesson in my error and then let it go, but like many young children, this concept exceeded my grasp.

Later, as a young man, moments of strategic reflection still eluded me; all I could do was daydream. I knew I was supposed to be thinking and contemplating, but my mind was blank. From my discussions with my parents and my teachers, I learned that many people from all walks of life lacked this skill. However, the ability to think your way through important decisions is essential. As I confessed my own ineptness to do so in high school, I corrected this in my college years by learning contemplation.

How Big is Your World?

How many people do you know who re-live the same week over and over? They watch the same television shows, make the same comments, and do the same things day in and day out. Their life is structured by their schedule at work, their schedule at home and their sleep schedule. There is no time for breaking the cycle, for thinking grand thoughts or actively working toward a brighter future. However, when you make contemplation a priority, you can find ways to incorporate it into your daily routine.

Recently, a client of mine retired. Bob was an office worker for a large corporation. Five days a week Bob worked the day shift, came home to watch the evening news at dinner, watched his favorite TV shows and, at bedtime, played the same music. For over 20 years his weekends were composed of lawn work, church and televised sporting events. Retirement shattered this structured life and led him to my office. Bob's complaint was that he did not know what to do with his life. When I suggested he do exactly what he wanted to do, he became more puzzled.

Bob was one of the many "baby boomers" who are entering retirement and finding themselves overwhelmed with too much free time. His world had been fairly small and very consistent – he never ventured from the safety of his job and home. And more to the point, he never contemplated his life, his role in the world and his goals. He was dismayed to discover how narrow his fundamental views were of the world. He knew very little about how other people lived in his own community and was vastly ignorant about lifestyles in foreign lands. Retirement removed his blinders and he was starting to see the true size of the world. Because it seemed much larger than his self-concept, he felt dwarfed. It was time for him to expand his worldview and his self-concept. It was time for him to learn about contemplation.

Once he realized that his tiny world provided only a glimpse of what the larger world had to offer, he became fascinated. Previously, he read his daily newspaper as a casual observer and glanced through his issues of *National Geographic* in the same detached manner. Now he had become a seeker; he really wanted to know about the lives of other people and was also searching for new options for himself. He began to see documentaries and his stacks of old magazines in an entirely new light. Through the printed words and his DVDs, he was meeting the people of distant lands and foreign cultures. He wanted to visit them. His mind became full of possibilities and amazing thoughts. His world was quickly expanding.

During our sessions, he talked with great enthusiasm about the other worlds he was discovering. It was as if he had been living on an island in a distant land. He had blindly followed the rules of job security instead of joy. He was a good man, but was rapidly realizing that he had settled for a very limited existence. He was learning how much more there was to life – and it was more than he ever imagined.

As he started to contemplate his life after retirement, I encouraged him to develop a regular practice of meditation. Combining meditation and contemplation together helped him quickly gain access to the voice of his own conscience. It would be that voice that would lead him to the next step in his life. As the weeks rolled by, his reading and his personal practices opened his eyes wider and wider. The freedom of retirement was no longer frightening and his life started to fill with wonderment and possibilities for the future. At our last meeting, he proudly displayed his newly acquired passport. Bob was ready to meet the world.

I Enter the Movie of My Own Life

As I stated earlier, my own admission ticket to the inner world of contemplation was thrust in my hand by Mary, the patient I described earlier in this chapter. Up until this woman's struggles showed me "the missing link," my life had been like a movie to me. I watched what happened in my life, but I did not feel like the main character and certainly not like the director. Thanks to Mary, that changed overnight. I left the audience. I became the star, the director and the producer of this magnificent film. I finally took charge of my life.

Contemplation helps you to start making connections, first one, then another, then a flood of insight and understanding about the relationship between your thoughts and actions. Life becomes very sequential to the astute observer and you begin to actively participate in the game. You become aware of the power of your seemingly irrelevant decisions or actions. These are the little daily choices that you never knew how much they could help or hurt your personal progress. Making these connections transforms your life. You become more hopeful as you see how your directed thinking starts to bring you a brighter, calmer, happier way of living. You become more protective of your determination as you wield this new sword of decision with care and skill. As your personal decisions and choices direct your own thoughts and actions, you gain a powerful feeling of freedom and power.

Thanks to contemplation, your life and your meditation no longer live in a passive state. Your life becomes a dynamic interaction guided by refreshing active wisdom. Other people in your life become important and are welcomed by you. Your own sense of satisfaction births the desire for serving and inspiring others. It is a natural expansion of your life to share your joy with others. To be happy, you must mold yourself into a person that shines and delights in making others shine. You begin to brighten the lives of those around you, and that joy cannot be compared to anything in this world. Some people try to make themselves look good by making others look worse, but such actions are never found in the lives of happy people.

> *Contemplation hones and refines your ability to listen to your conscience.*

MAKING PROGRESS

As your mind becomes stable and quiet, a multitude of thoughts, feelings and memories may come into your awareness. They are the reactions, reflections and insights that were easily displaced by the roar of your duties and desires. Buried among them is the voice of your conscience, the buddhi. Contemplation hones and refines your ability to listen to your conscience.

While learning to quiet your mind, it is helpful to understand how you trigger those occasional avalanches of thoughts and feelings. Contemplation awakens the subtle impressions in your mind. Without a thought, they cannot be activated. The subconscious mind can only be stirred by the conscious mind, even though this stimulus can be in the very subtle form of thought, fantasy or curiosity. That is why determination (willpower) is the key companion to contemplation. For, it is the strength of your willpower that can minimize any potential storm from the subconscious. All subtle impressions of the past lay dormant in the subconscious mind until something awakens them. Thus, it is essential that you contemplate (with full determination) on positive attributes that are contrary to the unhelpful tendencies that arise in your mind. This is the antidote to all negativity and fear that dominates the minds of many of my patients. Contemplation is a matter of gathering your courage and tapping into your inner strength that will allow you to ride out the powerful waves of emotions without beaching on the sand dunes of the past. In this process you may fail many times. Take those moments as lessons on how to be more skillful as you try again and again. Eventually, you will succeed.

No one can achieve freedom from fear through worldly actions alone. At the deepest level of your being, contemplation coupled with inner strength is the only solution. Your personal experience will eventually verify this fact. At some point you will discover the truth about your existence and identity. That discovery, that moment, will redress the entire landscape of your life. Beauty and consistency return as you view yourself and your world from a wholly integrated perspective. The knowledge you seek must wake you up and move you toward this experiential conclusion. Knowledge that is not functional and practical to your pursuit of lasting happiness is a burden best set aside for now. After all, this entire text is about your quest for happiness. Seek out valid, time tested knowledge. Study the lives of those who have achieved the happiness you are seeking. If possible, interview them and study with them. Let their success inspire you to complete your quest. Contemplate your strengths.

> *Knowledge that is not functional and practical to your pursuit of lasting happiness is a burden best set aside.*

STAYING ON TASK

Defining your core beliefs and your ultimate identity will help you stay focused on the task at hand. If you do not know yourself, you waste time defending yourself and chasing after tantalizing objects that will later disappoint you.

Your conscience is dying to have your attention and your ear. It will help guide your behavior and reactions to the people and events in your life. Your conscience will provide you with insights about you and your life. It acts as a bright light illuminating the darkest recesses of your mind. You will learn to navigate through the fields of memories and impulses by maintaining a constant awareness of both the goal of your journey and your identity.

AN INTRODUCTION TO CONTEMPLATION

During the practice of contemplation, you can and must be honest with yourself. It is a private time. Listen to yourself. Discover and define the difference between the fanciful noises of your mind and the inner voice that is you. Your goal is to hear and heed the voice of your conscience. Once you identify and listen to your conscience, then you can put the teachings of others into proper perspective. Things will begin to make sense. From that day forth, it becomes easy to select what is reasonable and meaningful in your life. You will no longer waste your time on activities that are not consistent with your goals.

> *Unexamined thoughts and actions will keep you helplessly repeating that which you no longer wish to do.*

Sit down. Contemplate the urgent issues of your life. Use the questions in the next paragraph to get you started. They are very broad questions with no right answer, just your opinion. Your answers will change over time. You may find great benefit from answering these questions on a weekly or monthly basis. Write your new answers before reviewing your opinions of last month.

Who am I?

What am I doing?

Why am I doing it?

What is the purpose of my life?

What do I want to achieve in my life?

What did I do in the past?

What were the outcomes of my past actions?

What did I learn from my past activities?

What actions helped me and what activities distracted me from my goals?

What mistakes did I make and how did I react to my errors?

Are the memories of past mistakes haunting or crippling my efforts today?

These contemplative questions help you understand your actions of the past, their results and how they can be used to guide your future actions. Unexamined thoughts and actions will keep you helplessly repeating that which you no longer wish to do.

Pinning your mind down on paper is very helpful. The power of the written word is a cultural and historical fact. When you document your goals in writing, it multiplies their power. Words are also specific and exact; your writing will help you clarify both your obstacles and your goals. Understanding the importance of your goals and the effort needed to achieve your goals is critical to your success.

> *"If you are really serious, put it in writing."*

CONTEMPLATE ON WHAT?

Contemplation means to reflect on yourself, your decisions and the events you have participated in or witnessed. I have never believed in coincidence or chance; my own philosophy is that everything happens for a reason. Have you ever noticed how the phone rings or the computer freezes just at that moment when you truly *need* an interruption — something to shake you loose from a downward spiral of thoughts or feelings? My conversations with Panditji continually catapulted me to new ways to view my life and life events and also aided in the further development of my contemplation techniques. As I was just learning contemplation, an event involving Panditji and a baby at 30 thousand feet gave me a lesson that I still reflect on today.

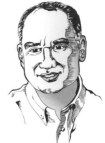

Pandit Rajmani Tigunait, Ph.D.

It happened years ago, when Karen and I were flying back from India on a crowded plane. Across the aisle sat Panditji and his wife. Ten rows ahead of us was an elderly Indian man, frantically trying to quiet a screaming infant in his care. After a good deal of time, this poor fellow's efforts continued to fail. Karen went up to him to offer her assistance.

Before I knew it, the thrashing, screaming child was now beside me in my wife's lap. Her gentle cooing did soothe the infant slightly, but only slightly. She had learned that the infant was from an orphanage, and that the gentleman's daughter in New York City had adopted this child and he was serving as the guardian and stork.

Finally, she handed the child to me to see if I could be of any assistance. I was not. However, Panditji, who had been watching this whole drama unfold, decided to intervene. His technique was clear, powerful and effective.

He leaned across the aisle, coming to within inches of the child's face. In a firm but kind voice, he commanded, "Life is a mountain, kick it into dust!" The child retorted with large eyes and a backward lunge, as if his words had struck her face with gale force. Then, her eyes brightened and she smiled. It was as if she knew that someone, in this case Panditji, understood her plight. Seemingly pleased with his acknowledgement, she became quiet and happy for the rest of the long journey to her new home and her new world.

Panditji knew that the baby girl had come from a difficult situation and now she, herself, must take charge of her life and conquer the challenges her birth had given her. No excuses and no pity, just encouragement to go do what has to be done in order to have a great life. She must kick the mountain of challenges that she will face until they crumble into dust.

It seemed that a few honest words that recognized this baby's upcoming challenges had shaken her loose from her downward spiral. Whether the infant experienced some change at the level of her soul, I do not know. Karen and I both saw a dramatic difference in her that was noticeably pleasant and serene for the rest of our trip. Many times in my life a single comment, a phrase in a book or a burst of inspiration brought forward an invisible force that would shake me loose. If you want to be free of misery, acknowledge those moments that can stop your freefall into gloom. Even today, I re-read certain books and re-live certain conversations over and over as reminders to take those interruptions seriously.

Over the years, my journal has become filled with simple statements and summaries that help me recall life-changing moments in my personal growth. They serve as a foundation for my contemplation.

"Life is a mountain, kick it into dust."

"How can a person be happy if he treats himself as his own worst enemy?"

"What other people think of you, is none of your business."

"Selfless service is an acquired taste."

"Self-esteem is a person's greatest wealth – and humanitarian service is the greatest form of worship."

"Be good, do good."

"Knowing that you can quit at any time, then why quit now?"

"Never delay a good thing."

What five phrases or comments guide your decisions and reactions each day? Take a moment and write them down. Do they lead you where you wish to go? If not, re-write them in a manner that will lead you somewhere good. Polish them with precision and kindness. Keep refining them or even rejecting them until you have a foundation that supports you and your loved ones. You can make your notes here:

1_____

2_____

3_____

4_____

5_____

CONCLUSION

The central core of this book has been clearly revealed in this chapter. I have spoken here with a clear and strong voice that some critics may see as dogmatic and even overpowering. Science is commonly that way. The sun is seen in the east every morning, it is not subject to a democratic vote. Likewise, as our society suffers from a weakened willpower that allows fear and doubt to dominate, yoga responds with clarity and exactness. Yoga science is verified every day through practice. This experiential verification leads you to both victory and validation.

Through the grace of my teachers and my own experience, I am able to share with you techniques that will help anyone who applies them properly. I believe that very few people ever find a valid teacher because they don't know it is a real option. It is my hope that this book will encourage every reader to strive for self-improvement and attain greater health and happiness. It is often said that when the student is ready, the teacher will appear.

Resolve to find happiness within you now. Use the experiences of the sages and the testimony of your own scriptures to inspire your faith in your own efforts. Your own faith and resolve will help you gain experience of the truth within you. This becomes an internal reinforcing cycle that will continue to inspire you to achieve greater levels of insight and joy. It gives you the courage to turn away from the false hopes of materialism and find the truth of your being in the place where all limitations end.

The longing of your soul will set you on the path and keep you there until you realize your true identity. You will encounter a multitude of distractions and side trips, but keep going. It does not matter what your age or career may be, all that matters is a willingness to discover the truth about yourself. Your inner spirit manifests as that invisible force that keeps pulling you toward higher levels of self-understanding. You cannot ignore your body or your mind; instead befriend them and they will become your allies and companions on your journey home.

To assist your ability to hear the voice of your conscience, I have included in the Appendix B a very special contemplation practice. It is called, "There is no other." If you read and consider its message once a day for the next 11 days, I am confident that it will help you. Please take a moment and go to Appendix B.

CHAPTER SUMMARY

· Contemplation helps you endow your life with clarity and purpose. It will ensure that you gain wisdom and guidance from your life experiences and move forward in a positive direction rather than repeating aimless cycles of events.

· Contemplation is the art of skillfully guiding your internal dialogue in a manner that helps you reflect on who you are, what you are doing, why you are doing it, how you will do it and what you have learned from your past experiences.

· The subconscious mind needs to be stirred by some stimulus from the conscious mind in order to be activated. Contemplation, with full determination, on positive attributes and ideas will prevent unhelpful tendencies from arising in your mind.

ACTION ITEMS

· If you worship any particular god or concept of divinity, write down the positive attributes your concept of god has and do your best to imitate these.

· Answer the questions on page 257 of this chapter in writing.

· Choose five phrases, quotes, or helpful sayings from this book, or elsewhere, that you feel could help to guide your decisions and reactions on a daily basis.

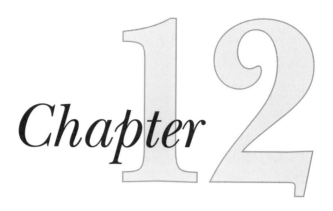

Chapter 12

Acquiring a Joyful Mind
The Philosophy of Meditation

A s a child, whenever I felt sad or had a scary dream, I ran to my parents for comfort. Today I see my adult patients running in much the same way. They run in many directions because they need reassurance on how to cope with their thoughts and feelings. Don't get me wrong: this is not a bad thing. Seeking help from others is an acceptable reaction and has become mainstream in our culture. In the 21st century we are open about our weaknesses and support groups dot the map. However, it was not always that way.

Let's leapfrog through a few milestones in psychotherapy. Only a few decades ago, mental health was a forbidden topic. During that era it was quite rare that anyone would ask for help. Some people drowned their unwanted thoughts in alcohol. Some talked about their thoughts with others, gathering opinions on how to react. Some quietly hid them, hoping that no one would notice that they were suffering in silence. It was a time of secrecy and we should all be glad it's over.

Interestingly, in ancient times, there was a different approach. Great saints and sages, appearing at different times and in different lands, instilled far healthier attitudes about mental health in their respective societies. These wise ones knew that unhappy people can spend so much time dealing with their thoughts and impulses that they have no time for life, love and laughter. Furthermore, they knew the power of the conscience and how to harness it. It was an age of meditation and self-reliance.

Nurturing and reassuring yourself is the methodology taught by the sages. It is the science and philosophy of meditation. It provides you with a safe and systematic way to examine and transform your own thinking patterns. Through meditation, you allow your thoughts to rise up for your inspection and then you organize them and skillfully redirect them. Meditation improves

> *An unhappy person can spend so much time dealing with their thoughts and impulses that they have no time for life, love and laughter.*

your ability to function at home, at work and at play. Remember that you are treading the path of health and happiness - everything you do can be transformed into an act of joy and understanding.

Ordinary people have ordinary problems -- and common problems can have common solutions. But special problems require special solutions. Most people go through life being part of the masses, blending in with the crowd rather than standing out. As you start to do a little more to improve your life than the ordinary person does, that small effort transforms your life from being ordinary to being "extra-ordinary."

An extraordinary life is lived between two extremes — the mountain of blessings and privileges and the mountain of challenges and strife. No longer settling for a life of quiet desperation, you vividly experience the fullness that each day brings. You will be able to balance these extremes in your practice of meditation.

Every day, set aside a few moments to maintain your self-selected perspective on how your day and life are progressing. As you initially become more inspired about the possibilities in your life, tiny personal flaws may seem larger than they really are. It is as if the tiniest stains in your mind are given more attention than they deserve. With time and meditation, you will easily understand how to maintain a proper perspective. When I talk with my patients and friends about this perspective, I start with the story of the grape juice stain.

Once upon a time, there was a blanket. It was a favorite blanket and the family found many uses for it. Over the years it became soiled and stained. Never thinking to wash the blanket, the family carried it with them on every outing and occasion. Then, one day, the youngest child spilled a small drop of grape juice on the blanket that years ago had been a brilliant white.

Fate had it that months after this latest spill, the family decided to launder the blanket. This decision caused the parents to look realistically at the blanket's condition. Mud and grime and interwoven debris kept them from placing the blanket in their new washing machine. Instead, they decided to hose the blanket off in the driveway. The water hose removed the caked mud, but the ground-in leaves and twigs did not stir from the forceful shower. The family next decided to soak the blanket in the bathtub. Quickly the water turned brown. Over and over they rinsed the blanket as the fragments of debris floated to the surface. Finally they decided to try washing the blanket in their new machine. The blanket was washed and dried. Out of the dryer came the fluffy white blanket and it appeared almost perfect . . . almost.

When they unfolded the blanket, everyone noticed that the tiny purple stain of grape juice remained. The blanket that used to be completely filthy and acceptable was no longer welcome because of the glaring presence of the small purple stain among the huge field of white. After weeks of missing his favorite blanket, the young child who had spilled the grape juice pulled the blanket from the closet. He demanded that the blanket become part of family life once again. Hearing his parent's displeasure at the stain, the boy suggested that they find a stain remover that would help the blanket regain its full glory.

You see, the ordinary wear and tear had been removed by ordinary means. However, the standard cleansing options were not enough to remove the purple stain. In their desire to please their child, the parents had to consult with experts in the textile industry. The expert advice was quickly heeded, yielding a wonderful result. The blanket had regained its purity and its place in the family picnics. Knowing how durable and resilient the blanket was, the family now used it daily — and the child was filled with delight.

> *Meditation will allow you to observe firsthand the nature of your mind and the nature of your self.*

This story is really the story of everyone. Like the blanket, we go everywhere and do everything. Over time, our mind, like the blanket, bears the strains and stains from years of use. It is only when we start to clean up our mind that we eventually discover a glaring stain in our health or personality that was previously hidden among the grayness of our life.

Removing the stains from your mind is the initial goal of meditation. It is possible to gently cleanse the dust and dirt from your mind in a manner similar to how the blanket was treated. In the proper environment, the debris from the past will simply float free. This initial process of cleansing and mending the mind and personality can be achieved by dietary changes, lifestyle adjustments, exercise and other methods as noted throughout this book. Meditation can also be a part of this initial process, but when the stain in the mind requires expert attention, that is when the combined efforts of meditation, contemplation and psychotherapy can yield amazing results. This triad of therapy will help you come to know your impulses and interests. However, meditation alone will allow you to observe firsthand the nature of your mind and the nature of your self.

> *The conscience is the home of wisdom, confidence, compassion and playfulness.*

In your practice of meditation, you will discover that there is a distinct difference between the mind and the self. For simplicity, the mind is composed of three parts: the ego, the memory and the flow of sensory data — including speech, hearing, touch and movement of the limbs. The self is defined as the conscience — that entity that's known to the poet as the voice of the heart, to the priest as the voice of the soul and to the intellect as the voice of reason. As the voice of the conscience is strengthened and discerned, you realize that your conscience is your true identity. When your mind is quiet, it is the conscience that comes forward. Meditation is the most effective method of allowing this experience to unfold.

Traditionally, the highest union - the union between mind and conscience - was called *yoga*. When this union occurs, the mind becomes the servant of the conscience instead of the master. This relationship – this union -- wields unlimited power as all internal conflicts (doubt, fear, anger, and greed) are quelled. The power of this experience arises from the freedom gained by no longer being a puppet to the whims and wishes of an inconsistent mind. The conscience is the home of wisdom, confidence, compassion and playfulness. You are finally able to take charge of your life because you have realized that you – the conscience – have always been in charge of your life. You can choose how you react to life events, including your own thoughts and feelings. You can choose what you want to do with your life. You are in charge because you are the only one who *can* be in charge.

The forging of this union is transformative at every level of your life. It is the first goal of all spiritual practices.

It took a long time for me to truly accept that the impulses in my mind do not have to be obeyed. I had been struggling to make the voice of my conscience louder and it seemed to be a frivolous pursuit. I knew that every time I sat for meditation my mind would try to hurry me through the process. This hurriedness was based in my mind wanting to please the senses by providing for them a constant variety of scenes and sensations. Finally, one day while sitting quietly, I halted this harassment caused by my mind. It was so simple that I laughed out loud to myself. I knew that my thoughts only had the power that I myself provided them. The moment I stopped being afraid of and fascinated with the mind's huge repertory of images and impulses was the moment my mind became quiet. It was my own fear and fascination empowering these thoughts. Everyone can learn to quiet their mind.

A few years ago I spoke to Panditji about a patient who I feared was canceling his psychotherapy appointments with his counselor. Panditji immediately and powerfully said, "He is a good man. If he is busy trying to be strong on his own, why should he go see that doctor? What is wrong with modern psychology? Why can't they let people be strong on their own? Just because they have the habit of always wanting people to lean on them, this does not mean your patients have to have this sickness of leaning." My mind drifted away from Panditji's voice. I was so embarrassed. In fearing for the welfare of my patient, I had forgotten that there was no reason to be afraid.

This man, like everyone, has the power to no longer be dominated by the impulses of his mind.

Panditji continued. "Let him be strong. He is a strong man; he does not need to lean on others. It is more important for a person to try to stand up and be strong than to never try at all." In a most quiet voice he said, "If his strength is not sturdy enough, gently guide him back into therapy, but if he is actually announcing to you his graduation from the neediness of outside counselors, then it means that he is becoming more aware of his conscience - the best guide and therapist."

While I am writing these words based on my own experience, I would never have developed an ability to write without a multitude of English and grammar teachers. Likewise, an external teacher is commonly needed to help one recognize and gain access to the voice of their own conscience. It seems that this solution of self-realization is so close to us that we, ourselves, are blind to it. Studying with Panditji continually removes my own blinders and expands my paradigm about how the world works. From my own study and reflection, I am convinced that the potential of the human psyche is unlimited and untrained.

Through meditation, the field of my own mind became my testing ground for these newfound insights and techniques. My experiments today are as exciting and challenging to me as they were almost 30 years ago. Try being happy on a really bad day. That's what I did. Every failure and every success was equally fascinating and useful. Sometimes I foolishly challenged a strong, deep-seated habit in my mind and quickly fell from grace. But with a sportsman-like attitude, I gradually learned to confront only the impulses, memories or fears that were well matched to my inner abilities. And game time was 6 a.m. – the time of my morning meditation.

During my meditation I achieved success in the lower ranking areas of my mind and I gradually promoted myself to the arena of more dominating and more unwanted habits. The more I learned, the more I wanted to meditate. When meditation is an active process that builds your self-confidence and self-understanding, then no one will need to motivate you to sit down and meditate.

The story of the blanket with the grape juice stain has always been a vivid lesson for me. Outside of meditation, my progression of self-transformation was quickened by my conversations with mentors and by my efforts to compassionately guide my students and clients who were fixated on their tiniest stains of insignificance.

Each person's suffering became a modern day example of the same suffering that I experienced in the past. I found tremendous value in the stories of my students and clients. I learned to ask direct questions that revealed a clear depiction of their weaknesses and strengths. The more vivid the problem, the more obvious the solution became to both of us. These conversations became sacred - their time of personal despair became the key that helped them regain their righteousness and virtue. Their failures and eventual victories inspired us both. Meditation was their hall of victory.

> *When meditation is an active process that builds your self-confidence and self-understanding, then no one will need to motivate you to sit down and meditate.*

For over 20 years I have had the privilege of guiding and clarifying individuals' experience from a wide variety of meditative traditions. Regardless of the origin of their training in meditation, they are all subject to the same universal guidelines. Those who have been actively meditating for years want to know why they are not achieving the results they are seeking. And those who have never meditated, but want to manage their stress more effectively, are filled with questions about why meditation is so important. Both practitioners and non-practitioners of meditation are seeking one thing: happiness.

Here is the bottom line: you have to be able to live with yourself. Regardless of your marital status or your occupation, there will be times when you will be physically alone. Those are the moments when you get to spend some extra time with your mind. Depending upon the relationship you have with your mind, your moments of solitude will either be pleasant or unpleasant.

> *Depending upon the relationship you have with your mind, your moments of solitude will either be pleasant or unpleasant.*

Now, if the last two sentences piqued your curiosity, then you are probably ready to learn how to meditate. It is a fantastic voyage.

Imagine that you are going to embark on a magical tour of the inner workings of your life. On this voyage you will view the precursors to every success and delight that you experience. And you will view from concept to creation, how problems are formed that impair your self-confidence and compassion. Your journey will be in real time, allowing you to immediately feel the consequences of these inner workings. On this voyage you will also be provided with expert guidance from a variety of sources, including your meditation teacher, sacred texts and your own conscience. This expertise will offer you tips, techniques and insights on how to increase your joy, productivity and kindness. This is the voyage of meditation. You get to see the inner workings of your mind, up close and personal. That is why you must thoroughly understand the philosophy of meditation and the tools of meditation before you leave the "home port" of the external world.

Every year meditation is becoming more popular. It is in vogue at many levels of society in America and abroad. According to *Newsweek* (Aug. 29th, 2005), approximately 30 percent of Americans now say they practice meditation regularly. While more people are practicing meditation, I wonder what they are actually doing. To simply meditate aimlessly, without acquiring a joyful mind, is too easy and too common. You need a philosophy and time-tested techniques to succeed at this goal – the real goal of meditation.

While there is no certifying body for teachers of meditation, there is a living tradition of meditators that stands from the earliest of times. You may find great value in reviewing the literature of this science – the *Vedas, Upanishads and Yoga Sutras*, the *Bhagavad Gita, Tripura Rahasya* and the *Puranas*. These are the published "scientific journals" of the meditative tradition.

Many of these texts are records of conversations between students and teachers. In the days during which they were written, the only salvation from despair and inner turmoil was guidance from a person who had attained the very goal you were pursuing. It was a time and a place where students respectfully laid their confusion and misguided deeds at the feet of their teacher. In that moment, the student immediately sensed the unconditional love of his teacher and only in that atmosphere could he feel safe and secure enough to learn how to resolve the mortification and consequences of his own actions. These powerful conversations of transformation, healing and growth have been recorded and recited throughout history. These living stories bring to life the healing relationships between parent and child, student and teacher, guru and disciple. In many parts of the world, this kind of loving relationship is still kept alive and is still being recorded in stories saved through the printed word.

Thus far in this book, I have shared with you the secrets and short-cuts that enable you to maximize joy and minimize misery. These methodologies will help you learn to identify more with your conscience than your mind, and eventually, you will merge the two. At the moment that this union is forged, all internal conflicts will cease and all personal confusions will end. Until this revelation dawns, you will need a guide. Until a living teacher appears, there are great conversations preserved in the spiritual literature that helped my patients and will help you. For what my patients were seeking is what you are seeking — happiness.

These stories continue to live because they address every issue and every dilemma that you could ever encounter throughout your entire life span. Every culture and every time period has recited tales blending history, technique and inspiration to their loved ones.

In December of 2000 I visited a tiny village of fisherman living along the Ganges River outside of Allahabad. Seeing a small group of Westerners, the villagers gathered to greet us. Within moments, the village leader appeared, along with his council of musicians, inviting us to sit down and listen to the story of their town. They sang with power and delight about their mother - the river Ganges - and how she sustains their life by providing them with food, water and jobs. In the next hour, through the graciousness of an interpreter, I learned that their musical stories were filled with advice on ecology, respect, faith, relationships, honor and courage. There were historical facts, spiritual lore and an overwhelming gratitude chorused together with rhythm and dance. All the children were eager to embrace and recite the songs of their village. It was a symphony of timeless love.

Today we no longer gather around a community fire to share our dreams and recite the story of our tribe. We meet in coffee houses or online chat rooms to recite jokes from our favorite television shows and tales of our favorite rock stars. The oral tradition of knowledge today is commonly limited to local gossip, nationalistic pride or fractured theologies that separate us from one another instead of unifying us all. We listen to iPods, satellite radio and television instead of speaking for ourselves and sharing the tale of transformation within our lives and the lives of our family. However, times are changing.

Teenagers now put their private thoughts online for all to read. They use the Internet to log the entries of their diary and they blog the news of their family to the world. The search for intimacy of thought and community is returning full force. Self-reflection is returning.

For many of my patients, it was their journals of private thoughts that led them to seek out instruction in meditation. Putting your thoughts and feelings into written words requires you to search and perhaps struggle for the right words that accurately convey your message. This forces you to clarify the true nature of your experience and your personal evaluation of that moment. Capturing your life on paper commonly reveals the answers you are seeking. Do not be afraid to express yourself in your own private manner. Sometimes the purpose of fear is to prevent questioning. Any fear that is questioned effectively will cease to exist.

Meditation allows you to safely examine and question your fears. This gentle and objective examination will lead you to a deeper understanding of yourself – a self that is free of fear and guilt, shame and doubt. Meditation polishes your mind, allowing you to see the brilliance of love, compassion and wisdom. A patient once asked me how to surrender guilt. I told her that before you can surrender anything, you must clearly understand that you will be gaining much more of what you truly want by the process of surrender. You must realize that by giving up guilt, you will gain far more joy. Likewise, you will give up activities that have never led you to peace. You will never find time to meditate until you find an activity that never works for you and then surrender that moment in exchange for time to learn meditation. It is a gradual process.

In time, your own story will be one of triumph and joy.

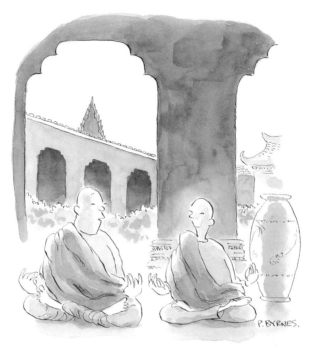

"Are you not thinking what I'm not thinking?"

THE OBJECT OF MEDITATION

The outcome of meditation, which is the process of paying attention, is dependent upon the object of the meditation. If your meditation posture is not comfortable, your mind may meditate on the uncomfortable sensations. If your mind is angry and upset, your meditation experience may be limited to the repetitive drone of the topics that have upset you. The meditative literature of the past recommends that teachers of meditation today should encourage the object of meditation to be a mantra.

A mantra is a sacred awakened sound that guides and protects the meditator from the subtle unhelpful impulses in his or her mind. The mantra also awakens and quickens your awareness of positive qualities within you that may not currently be in your awareness. Cultivating your mind with the richness of courage, love, responsibility and insight allows you to be productive and delightful throughout your entire life. Your mantra guides you through all troubled times by revealing the insights and advice of your own conscience. Eventually the mantra leads you to a state of silence and satisfaction. In that culminating moment you experience the true nature of your own identity – the state of self-realization. The ultimate cure for all fear and stress dwells in this well of silence deep within you. To go there is to know the joy that answers all questions. Mantras unlock all doors and lift you over every hurdle as you seek out the silence within you.

Soham, pronounced so-hum, is the first mantra of a meditator. It has the very rare quality of flowing with your breath. When you inhale, you silently recite the sound of 'so.' During exhalation, recite the sound of 'ham.' Most mantras are independent of the breath, but not *soham.*

This mantra comes awakened and ready to use. It does not require formal initiation by a teacher or any external rituals. Just simply sit down and bring the mantra forward into your awareness. For those who are prepared for a more advanced practice of meditation, seeking out a teacher in the meditative tradition is recommended. If no teacher can be found, there are two other mantras that are also available to you in the public domain. These mantras, Gayatri and Maha Mrityunjaya, are also immediately available to you. They have a rich history dating back to the dawn of time. Here is an explanation of these mantras.

The Gayatri mantra is:
Om Bhur Bhuvah Svah
Tat savitur varenyam
Bhargo devasya dhimahi
Dhiyo yo nah prachodayat

The translation of this mantra is, "I meditate on the radiant and most venerable light of the divine from which issues forth the triple world – the bhur, bhuvah and swah – earth, space and heaven. May the divine light illuminate and guide my intelligence."

This mantra is traditionally called the Mother of the Vedas. The practice of this mantra enabled the sages to receive the revelation of all other mantras. This mantra calms mental noises, washes off karmic impurities, purifies ego, sharpens the intellect and illuminates the inner being with the light which flows directly from the source.

The Maha Mrityunjaya mantra is the means for attaining victory over death, disease, and sickness. The word "maha" means great, "mrityu" means death, "jaya" means victory. This is a healing and nourishing mantra, cultivating the healing power within.

This is the mantra:
Om Tryambakam yajamahe
Sugandhim pushti vardhanam
Urvarukamiva bandhanan
Mrityor mukshiya mamritat

The translation of this mantra is: "I meditate on and surrender myself to the Divine Being who embodies the power of will, the power of knowledge and the power of action. I pray to the Divine Being who manifests in the form of fragrance in the flower of life and is the eternal nourisher of the plant of life. Like a skillful gardener, may the Lord of Life disentangle me from the binding forces of my physical, psychological and spiritual foes. May the Lord of Immortality residing within free me from my death, decay and sickness, and unite me with immortality."

You may not notice an instantaneous transformation from reciting these mantras, but their effect is immense and everlasting. The process of purification with mantra meditation begins in the deep subconscious and gradually pervades all aspects of your personality. You become new and fully transformed from inside out. According to the sages, there are two ways you can overcome obstacles to your spiritual awakening. The first method is to clear away the hurdles by overcoming your weaknesses and consequently gaining inner strength. The second method is to clear away the hurdles by making the strong part of yourself even stronger and consequently attaining freedom from weakness.

The Gayatri mantra uses the first method – it clears away the hurdles by overcoming weaknesses. The Maha Mrityunjaya mantra which is mainly used for healing, uses the second method. It clears away the hurdles by making the strong part of ourselves even stronger. The Gayatri mantra focuses on cleansing, while the Maha Mrityunjaya mantra focuses on nourishing. Ultimately, you achieve the same goal.

Proper pronunciation of all mantras is very important. You are welcome to request an audio CD of these mantras from my office. You can reach me online at www.AliveandHealthy.com.

Once a mantra has been received, the student of meditation starts to dedicate a self-selected time to regularly meditate on his mantra. A consistent daily practice of meditation will gradually lead you to true self-understanding and self-transformation. You can easily understand and experience meditation. Eventually you will match the experiences of the great meditators.

Let's meditate right now.

Bring your awareness to your forehead, the area between your two eyebrows. Start with your awareness there as you gently close your eyes and begin breathing in a smooth, rhythmic fashion through your nose. As your breath becomes smooth and continuous, become aware of your mantra. Remember the sound of "soham" and let it begin to blend in with your breath. Remember the sound of "so" during inhalation and the sound "hum" during exhalation. Let these two sounds soothe and massage your breath.

Hear the sound of "soham" in the sanctuary of your mind. Silent to the world, but within you a cacophony builds of spiritual awakening and renewal. As your mantra guides you deeper within, occasionally thoughts and ideas will surface. Witness them as they rise and dissolve. There is no need to get involved with thought patterns.

Meditation is your time to practice dealing with your own mental tendencies and impulses. When you disconnect yourself from your external relationship with your senses, it is only natural that the stored impressions in your mind will come forward. That is why solitude can be either pleasant or tormenting, based upon the skill an individual has in dealing with his or her mind. It is a learned skill. Solitary confinement to the prisoner is hell, but to the meditator it is heaven. It is only a difference of skill levels.

Give your mantra a higher priority than the thoughts, feelings and memories arising within. Do not allow the thoughts to affect you. Continue to breathe and keep the mind focused on the mantra. After 10 to 15 minutes, gradually conclude your meditation. Take a few moments to enjoy the calm stillness of your meditation.

Stillness in meditation will give you physical delight. Even if you are pretending to meditate it will help. Try to understand the conscious part of your mind - it is your constant companion. Learn to refine your entire mind (both the conscious and subconscious parts) by gently training yourself to be still. You will stumble many times, but if your goal is clear, providence will guide you. All problems of stress are created and cured by your breathing mechanism. Keep breathing and the stress will lessen. Soon it will be gone.

You may want to track your progress in a diary. By writing down your observations once a week, you will clearly see how your life is transforming. It is the questions you ask yourself that reveal these data. Did thoughts surface during meditation? Did important thoughts and images come to your mind that you had forgotten? What happened when you guided your awareness back to your mantra?

There were times when I needed to pause and write down certain thoughts during my meditation time. I was so convinced that these thoughts were too important to forget. By quickly writing them down, I purged them from my mind and my meditation became deeper. This would usually happen in the first few minutes of meditation.

Initially it may take you several minutes for your mind to calm down. As this happens, your awareness of your mantra becomes more dominant than the chatter of your mind. When this occurs, notice how calm and quiet your body has become. If your body is restless, you may need to travel through your body and settle down each major area. For instance, you can give your shoulders permission to fall away from your ears. Instruct your abdomen to rise and fall with each breath in a soft and rhythmic manner. Tell your facial muscles to release any expression being held and allow your face to feel quiet and relaxed. You may feel some gurgling and movement in your digestive system as tension is released, allowing your foods and fluids to progress through your intestines.

In meditation you will experience how much your mind has to say and directly observe the qualities of the mind's content. Acquiring a joyful mind is an inward journey that allows you to examine your own strengths and weaknesses without fear or regret. There is no need to hide your discoveries, but it is important to develop a philosophy that allows you to silently accept the contents of your mind as you guide your awareness deeper. Self-protective mechanisms are much more draining than they are supporting. In time you will learn to only store the impressions of your deeds that are selfless and kind in your mind. Do not dwell on other activities because they are usually not worth remembering. Delight, joy and happiness are the fruits of selfless actions.

Don't let your mind worry. Worry creates a hell inside you. The sages claim that worry is a living cremation that is much more painful than the cremation of the physical body. Many things in the mind can distract you. Act like a great swimmer who reaches forward and pushes the water behind. Likewise, you can push your thoughts behind you and continue to move ahead. If a swimmer pulls the water toward himself, he will stop moving and may drown. Your memories and distractions during meditation can become heavy weights that can drown your meditation experience if you are not alert. There is value in learning how to forget and how to unlearn. Parents and children alike can learn these skills.

To the meditator, everything in life becomes a means to joy. Taming the senses is much like taming a wild horse. A wild horse that hurts you once in a while is much better than a weak, starved horse - so learn to be a good rider. Transform the horse into a strong and obedient companion and then complete your journey. You can place more emphasis on transformation than on restraint. Transform the dark, heavy horse of the mind into a swift, bright, agile horse of joy.

❀   ❀   ❀

Chapter Summary:

- *The practice of meditation will allow you to observe firsthand the nature of your mind and the nature of your self (your conscience) and discover that there is a sharp difference between the two.*

- *The literal meaning of meditation is the process of paying attention. What you pay attention to, or the object of your meditation, will determine the results you experience. Using a mantra as an object of meditation will help prevent you from wasting your time by meditating on discomfort in your body or emotions that you may be feeling.*

- *When meditating, thoughts will arise. It is important to let these thoughts come and go without becoming disturbed by them. It is better to focus on increasing your awareness of your mantra than to try to suppress other thoughts.*

ACTION ITEMS:

- *Keep a journal of your private thoughts and feelings, and see whether this practice provides you with any insights or clarifications in your life.*

- *Choose a regular activity that you engage in now, that is either unhelpful or unnecessary in your life and replace it with time for learning to meditate.*

- *Practice meditation on the soham mantra as described in this chapter and keep a journal of your experience.*

❀   ❀   ❀

You can download my free eBook, Meditation: The Inward Journey, *for "How-to-tips" on meditation at <u>www.AliveandHealthy.com</u>*

❀   ❀   ❀

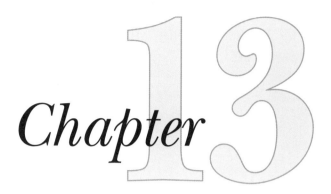

Chapter

Discovering Our Sacred Link
Establishing a Fellowship with Your Friends, Family and Community

As my meditation practice continued, my desire for fellowship grew. It was different from before. In the past I wanted constant company or activity because I feared stillness and got lost in silence. As I separated my identity from my inner mixture of emotions and thoughts, I felt a sense of security and relief. The experience piqued my curiosity about who I was. I wanted more time with me and I wanted more time with others who knew of these experiences. This was the fellowship I was seeking. My desire grew every day.

I learned to meditate in high school, but had no peer group support or guide. By the time I finished college, my inner longing to know myself and my desire for greater instruction was a full-time occupation. I kept feeling myself being pulled toward teachers and experiences that would fill in some of the blanks. I was looking for other pieces to the puzzle that would help me make sense of my life and understand my relationships with others.

Swami Rama spoke about how we should not work for ourselves but for the welfare of others. It made sense to me. I knew that self-lessness was the admission price for self-understanding. And understanding yourself is what everyone is seeking at a conscious or subconscious level. I had to find a way to blend my inner exploration with service to others. If I did it with the right attitude, both actions could catapult me to the goal. It took longer than I had planned. Although, in truth, I had never given myself a deadline, but when you grow up in an "instant on, instant off" world, the concept of delayed gratification seems archaic and frustrating. I wanted happiness immediately.

Gradually I became aware of the momentum of my own habits – some were pulling me toward my goals and some were dragging me away from them. For the unhelpful momentum to wear off, it was going to take some time, maybe years, unless I took a short-cut.

> *A good teacher knows how to entertain the student while nature takes its course.*

Clinging to old behaviors that disappoint you simply slows your journey to self-transformation. You have to ask yourself: Do you want to transform your life like a log rotting in the forest? Or do you want to transform yourself like a log thrown on a bonfire?

I chose the bonfire approach.

TURNING UP THE HEAT

I continually strengthened my refrain from all short-term substitutions and medications that would distract me from my goal of happiness. That really increased the fire. My friends and colleagues would medicate themselves with alcoholic beverages, over-socialization and spectator sports. Others filled their time with gambling or workaholic behaviors based in aquisition of wealth and competition. My approach was different. I was willing to experience every thought and feeling that my mind could conjure up. If I was heading off course, I wanted to be the first to know. I was living in the bonfire. On occasion I had to jump out of the fire, only to return another day.

As I struggled to understand myself, I simultaneously struggled to help others. I believe that only to the extent that I can help to free you from your bondage, do I purchase the right to free myself. This idea pounded in my head and heart. It gave the *golden rule* greater power and clarity as if there were no way to escape helping my fellow man. Poets and preachers urge all of us to uplift our community by lighting the flame of love in ourselves *and* in others. I could feel the spark starting to glow. I did not know how, but I knew I had to help.

My father used to say, "Remember what the old man said, 'If I had to do it all over again, I would ask for help.'" I have always been willing to play as a team member, but now I needed a real coach. I did not want to burn out. The pangs of joy and sadness were intense.

FINDING A MENTOR

Every skilled master of every trade was once an apprentice,
and every teacher once a student.

For my entire life I have needed teachers. From my youth, I realized my happiness was linked to the happiness of others and as a teenager I began searching for teachers who could help me learn how to help others.

At different stages of growth you need different mentors. When you learned the alphabet you didn't need the help of a college professor, you needed your first-grade teacher. Later, as an adult, you found mentors in the form of books, CDs, DVDs and seminars. As you grew and refined your process of self-transformation, you probably sought personalized instruction from someone who knew what you needed to know. From coaches to counselors to clinics, we seek guidance from experts.

You know that you will have to walk for yourself, but it helps to have someone show you how to take those first steps. And this was true in my life as well. Everyone wanted to be my teacher – and my parents, upon seeing my dilemma, pointed out that I must be cautious not to become too gullible. In my high school years alone I blazed through a multitude of teachers and techniques.

> *It is said that when the student is ready, the teacher will appear.*

It was the 1970s and self-transformation was the buzzword. Transactional Analysis training, volunteering at my local courthouse, community service through my church and becoming an instructor for the Red Cross gave me hundreds of contact hours with leaders in my community before my 18th birthday. Every moment seemed to be a lifetime of learning from these events. I am forever grateful to everyone who let me become a part of their mission.

As I saw value in community service, I continued to see the need to learn about how to live with myself. It was not an automatic condition. I did not know how to respond to myself when my own mistakes disappointed me. I knew if I wanted to achieve happiness in my life that I needed to find someone who had achieved happiness in their life. I was on fire and I didn't even know what was burning.

I think my initial approach to self-transformation through humanitarian service could best be defined as the "Ready-Fire-Aim" approach. At times, my exuberance jump-started my actions without pausing to take aim. I was going to change the world and improve myself no matter what. But I had no idea where to begin.

I needed the private coaching of an expert - a happiness expert, whatever that meant. It had to be someone who could help me now, and then let me graduate to higher levels of learning and the teachers of that knowledge. The purpose of an external teacher is to introduce you to the internal teacher within you - your purified conscience. This is the litmus test for true teachers – they must inspire you and encourage you to become more independent, to think independently and to assume greater levels of responsibility than you ever dreamed. Your capacity can be stretched and expanded, exceeding your wildest imagination. A true teacher forces you to grow in the most loving and deliberate manner.

Practice Makes Perfect

My patients repeatedly tell me how hard they are "working on themselves." Depending upon their mood and the moment, their task may be described as overwhelming or easily achieved. Making a New Year's resolution is not hard to do, but keeping the resolution *is* hard.

When you set your plans for the future, think like a master. Before you can master your emotions, you must feel like a master. When you perform your actions like a slave, then all you are doing is working. But when you perform your actions like a master, then there is a graciousness and a selflessness that greases your actions and activity. When you have no anxiety about the outcome of your actions, then the activity can transform you. But when you are only afraid of what others will think, then once again all you are doing is working. If you can easily change your plans and start over on your biggest project, then you are behaving like a master. If change is painful and criticism hurts you, then you are only working. As my patients learned to "work on themselves" as a master, they greeted every change and challenge with delight.

Practice does lead to perfection, but to be perfectly angry or disappointed is not the goal. Use all of your resources to stay inspired and continue to strive toward your goals. As you achieve your goals, they will expand and the possibilities will become unlimited.

I have never seen this in writing, but I want you to know this rarely mentioned fact. You are not interested in a flimsy temporary solution, you want solid long-lasting transformation. To attain this (and you can), each step or two along the way will need time to be assimilated into your life and breath. Too many times people tell me the same story with feelings of failure and disgust. The story is always the same. "I started taking yoga classes and I really loved it. But about eight weeks later, work got really busy and I had to stop going to class. Several months later I finally got back to class and life was grand for several months. Then my mother became ill and I have not been able to get back to class for almost a year now. I feel so bad about this."

In that story you could replace the phrase "yoga class" with any class or activity that fosters personal growth. When you start to change at core levels of your life, issues and situations that you need to pay attention to will surface quickly and powerfully. Thus, in this story about the yoga student, her "distractions" were subtly related to her progress. To build a firm foundation of peace within you, all levels of your life have to come into balance. That is why it takes many years for most of us to achieve a solid inner core and outer core of stability in our life. But when you finally get there, you will be standing on the Rock - elevated, steady, inspired and fully understood.

When you get involved in your own process of healing, I promise you will be pleased with the results. Participation in your health and happiness provides you with an indomitable sense of freedom and self-esteem. It frees you from the shackles of dependency and fear. No longer will you worry about losing your health or happiness, because you know all the essential ingredients to create it all over again.

The World Game Can Be Played at Home

When John Lennon sang, "Imagine there's no heaven," he was not trying to ignite religious or philosophical debates over what awaits us in the afterlife. Instead, he was making a simple and profound plea to all of mankind. We can squander the present, waiting for something better to come in the future, or we can make the world we are living in here and now as wonderful as possible. Why wait for heaven? Or simply put, never delay a good thing. Those who are full of love and compassion create heaven wherever they go. All of us strive to become this type of person. Surrounding yourself with others who emanate goodness will change your life and theirs.

You don't have to wait for the whole world to change. Transformation begins on an individual level and expands from there. As individuals transform, families, neighborhoods, cities, states and nations will follow. We learn by example. Many of our behaviors are merely imitations of something we have seen before. Therefore, provide the best example you can for others to imitate. In this way, one person at a time, the world will begin to discover the sacred link that unites us all – allowing the flower of humanity to blossom and unfold.

> *Transformation begins on an individual level and expands from there.*

Years ago Karen and I were walking with Panditji on a footpath outside of Rishikesh, India. Our pleasant stroll was interrupted by an astonished outburst from Panditji. We were walking through a beautiful valley when all of a sudden we encountered a pile of litter and trash covering the trail. "There you have it!" roared Panditji, pointing at the garbage. "Send an ignorant person to heaven and he will turn it into hell."

We continued on our walk, thinking about what Panditji had said. Only a few moments had passed when he suddenly halted and turned in our direction. Speaking in a much softer tone he said, "But if you send a wise person to hell, he will turn it into heaven." Our walk continued. Karen and I looked at each other as we both silently re-peated what we had heard: "Send an ignorant person to heaven and they will turn it into hell. But send a wise person to hell and he will turn it into heaven." We looked up. Panditji had stopped again. Now greeting us with his arms extended, he whis-pered, "If you wish, get really, really strong, ask for the privilege to go to hell... and turn it into heaven."

> *"If a nation expects to be ignorant and free, in a state of civilization, it expects what never was and never will be."*
> THOMAS JEFFERSON

His words were coming from the future. We did not know it then, but Panditji was forecasting our future. Ten years later global warm-ing, extreme poverty, biodiesel and AIDS would become the focus of our lives. Where there is drought, devastation, disease and despair, we want to help.

There is a wake-up call sounding around the globe. The sufferings of humanity and the planet itself are now becoming calls to action for every citizen and school child. We can no longer remain in a state of ignorance about global warming and other species-threatening behaviors.

BUILDING A BETTER WORLD THROUGH ACTION

For Karen and I, our travels to India became the spark to work for the betterment of others. It was definitely a bonfire approach and it was fueled by the poverty and destitution that we witnessed. All of us reach this point where the spark ignites and helping others becomes the fuel to help us attain our own goals. As your self-concept broadens, the welfare of others becomes more important.

All of us eventually gravitate toward the people and the opportunities that can help us achieve our goals – both lofty and mundane. There is no need to abandon your friends or family, but you must recognize that the only constant in life is *change*. As you and your mind become more supportive of your self-selected goals, the environment in which you live and work will gradually rise up to support you. Finding that support has become easier than ever. You can create a network of helpful people in your life by going on-line, by joining weekly classes or attending seminars. You can visit with these peers and mentors not just in person, but also through email, telephone, text messaging, instant messaging and so on. Your community is out there waiting for you. Go say hello.

As you can see in this chapter, I am expanding the concept of happiness to a higher level. When the forefathers of America wrote about "life, liberty and the pursuit of happiness," they were asking the citizens of their new nation and the world at large to reconsider the goals of

> *Praying for peace –*
> *even demanding peace*
> *– is not as powerful as*
> *living it.*

humanity. They saw this to be essential to the formation of a more perfect union. A much older document, the Vedas, expounds on yoga as *skillful living*. The Vedas state that yoga, or union, will come when you perform your actions skillfully in harmony with all forms of life. This synchronicity of goals and actions leads to a sustainable future. When all the individuals, cultures and nations of the world begin performing their actions skillfully, peace and prosperity will reign. This is the sacred link that binds us together. The longing for that connection dwells in you, as it dwells in me.

A huge component of skillful living comes down to how we treat ourselves and others. As we start to embrace diversity at the cultural and governmental levels, global policies will shift for the better. Governments will start to actively make peace and prosperity a priority. Someday, there will be a Department of Peace in every government and a Secretary of Peace in each president's Cabinet. We can initiate these changes now. You can inspire your government to create these positions, and to fill them with leaders who will bring peace within and promote peace and prosperity to other countries. If the great countries of the world would commit the same amount of effort and resources that they currently reserve for war into actively creating peace and prosperity, then everything could change quickly. Our behavior at the individual level can powerfully shift the collective behaviors of a nation. Praying for peace - even *demanding* peace - is not as powerful as *living* it.

Do not expect a democratic leader to be more generous or more peaceful than the citizens he or she serves. In every democracy the health and mindset of the citizens determine the actions and attitudes of their leaders. Good intentions are not enough. Many people have good intentions and yet there is still suffering in the world. Good intentions should be put into action. We must make a little more effort to greet and embrace the forces of good works. We cannot force others to change but we can change ourselves and become an example to the world. In the immortal words of Gandhi, "Be the change you wish to see in the world." With this attitude, Gandhi truly did change the world. Do not underestimate your impact.

The pure goodness and determination seen in the actions of Gandhi may seem like a lofty standard in which to hold yourself. There are, however, benchmarks along the way that you can aim for, as well as methods and guidelines for working toward true skillfulness in your interactions with others. Ask yourself everyday:

How much patience have I cultivated for my family members, friends and co-workers? How much sensitivity do I have toward the problems of others? How easily am I disturbed or angered by others? How do I respond to insult and injury from others?

Every great civilization has handed down guidelines for how to treat others. These guidelines consistently center on love, compassion and generosity toward all of mankind. Buddha said, "Hatred never ceases by hatred, but by love alone is healed. This is the ancient and eternal law. Like a caring mother holding and guarding the life of her only child, so with a boundless heart hold yourself and all beings."[32] The Gospel According to Matthew says, "Love your enemies, bless those who curse you, do good to those who hate you, and pray for those who spitefully use you and persecute you."[33]

In my own life I wanted to inspire all people, but I did not know how to respond to those who were not kind to me. In response to my dilemma I received the following loving instructions: All people are destined to be great and good some day. Some march toward their destiny while others occasionally get lost and distracted. Regardless of their current status, you share the same destiny.

> *Good intentions are not enough. Good intentions should be put into action.*

Whenever you see a wicked person, immediately say to yourself, "Someday he will be good." Whenever you see a good person, immediately say to yourself, "Someday he will be peaceful." Whenever you see a peaceful person, immediately say to yourself, "Someday he will obtain liberation from the tyranny of his mind." And, whenever you see a liberated person, simply bow your head.

Skillful interactions with others requires not just responding appropriately to those who are hostile, negative or displeasing to us in any way, but also responding appropriately to those who have been kind and helpful to us. Your personal lineage is filled with ancestors that many rarely acknowledge. Family is more than a bloodline, it is a legacy of culture refined for centuries to benefit you and those yet to come. This ongoing lineage has been preserved in the oral tradition as well as in the arts and music of every land. From a multitude of sources, I have recreated a tale that must be told.

According to legend, an ancient master imparted this advice to his son before sending him out into the world. He said: As you perform your actions, remember that you stand on the shoulders of your ancestors. Be grateful for all that you have inherited from them and think of what you can leave for those who come after you. You may think of your ancestors only as your direct blood relatives, but this is a limited view. You actually have four types of ancestors.

The first type is indeed your blood relatives. If it were not for them you would not be here today. They have given you everything about your body, from your flesh and bones down to your genetic make up. The parents of your bloodline have cared for and raised the children of your bloodline. The best way to serve these ancestors is to do what they have done for you. In your lifetime, provide another with the privilege of human life. Raise your own child or children with the utmost respect and care. In this way, you honor the sacrifices of your parents, grandparents, great grandparents and all those who preceded you in your family.

The second category of ancestors is made up of those who have provided our family lineage with material wealth, which includes employers, patrons and friends. Your relationship toward your employer is a sacred one. To honor our ancestors of this type, care for others to the best of your financial ability. When you become successful enough, employ those in need of work, give to those in need of charity. Keep only what you need for yourself. One who hoards more than he needs isolates himself from others and dishonors those who were generous enough to give to himself and his ancestors. Everyone, in some time and place, needed the guidance and charity of others.

The third category of ancestors is comprised of the scientists and teachers whose inventions and ideas made life easier. From the simplest inventions to the most fascinating and elaborate ideas, they passed on knowledge that saved many lives and gave us more time to care for one another. Do not take these gifts for granted. You can honor these ancestors by using the knowledge they have given us and expanding or improving upon their contributions. Use their knowledge and inventions in the most virtuous way - one that is conducive to the growth of mankind. The best way to honor these ancestors is to teach others. The virtue of contributing to the field of knowledge, through teaching others, exceeds all other good actions when done lovingly and selflessly.

The fourth and final category of ancestors is the forces of nature. Without air, sunlight or water, life simply could not exist. Nature serves all without discrimination or prejudice. The sun shines on the virtuous as well as the non-virtuous. Those who serve nature not only honor her, but they also leave a great legacy for generations to come. Consider the impact of your actions on nature. Consider what kind of planet you are leaving for future generations. Consider whether your actions convey the proper message of gratitude to the forces of nature. The water, air, soil and space carry the gross and subtle impressions of all of our actions. Therefore, contribute to the health of nature.

These are the four types of ancestors that have selflessly contributed to your world. None of them sought or seek your gratitude or praise. We honor and respect them all because we are grateful. We do our best to invest their gifts wisely to yield a greater return for future generations. Remember also that you are the ancestor of generations to come. Think always of your children, your children's children and all of the children to come thereafter. If it is within your capacity, provide them greater opportunities than your ancestors provided you. Be thankful for this great blessing of life.

CHAPTER SUMMARY

- *Before you can master your emotions, you must feel like a master. When you perform your actions like a slave, then all you are doing is working. But when you perform your actions like a master, then there is a graciousness and a selflessness that guides your actions.*

- *To build a firm foundation of peace within you, all levels of your life have to come into balance. That is why it takes many years for most of us to achieve that solid inner core and outer core of stability in our life.*

- *Good intentions are not enough. Good intentions should be put into action. We cannot force others to change, but we can change ourselves and become an example to the world.*

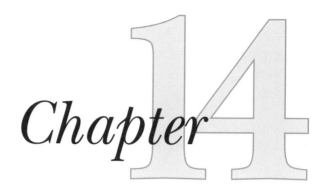

Love and Longevity

*"Love supersedes the regular laws of Nature,
including the law of karma."*
Pandit Rajmani Tigunait, PhD.

Thank you for traveling with me on this journey to joy. Within these pages I hope you have learned some useful strategies that will help you uncover the happiness within you. We know it is good to improve your diet, the benefits of exercise are countless, and the usefulness of prayer, contemplation and meditation are timeless. But it is unlikely that a single person could incorporate into his or her life all that has been taught in this book. I encourage you to gather even the smallest seed of a useful idea from any chapter, plant it in the fertile soil of your mind, and allow it to grow.

But beyond every strategy and technique mentioned within these

> *Every culture, tradition, and teacher throughout history has espoused this one perennial truth, "Love is the answer."*

pages lies something even greater, and I guarantee you that it will benefit you and yours. That something is *love*.

Writing this book has forced me to take a hard look at myself, my life, and the possibilities that yoga and spirituality can offer. My conclusion is simply this: there is very little that I have ever been able to do on my own or learn on my own. The first two decades of my life required the help, guidance, and teachings of many people to learn how to establish myself and navigate through life. I recall a student asking Swami Rama about the identity of the greatest yogi. The student had heard that the Sage Patanjali, the codifier of the Yoga Sutras, was the greatest yogi. The student asked Swami Rama if that was true. "No," replied Swamiji, "if it had not been for Patanjali's mother, he would never have attained these great achievements. His mother was the greatest yogi." And this summarizes my conclusion. If it were not

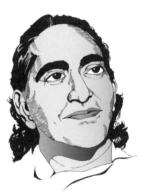

Sri Swami Rama of the Himalayas

for the love of my own parents, I would never have arrived. Therefore, love must be the answer.

The poets write that love is the answer, no matter what the question. But as for you and me — as we do our best to improve our diet, lifestyle, and relationships with a multitude of techniques — we would do well to remember that all the great sages declare that love supersedes everything. Love overrides the law of karma that you thought could never change.

If you can fall in love with life, if you can fall in love with your habits, your body and your personality, if you can fall in love with the people and animals you see around you, if you can do only that, you will find the happiness that is the goal of this simple book and the goal of all philosophies and theologies. And in that love you will find the fellowship of your neighbors and strangers alike. It is in that fellowship that I write these words to you.

BECOMING A CREATURE OF CHARM

Everything that has ever happened to you ... everything ... the good, the bad and the ugly ... has to be acceptable to you. To make the final leap to happiness, all you have to do is accept your entire life history and habits.

It is not possible to live a full life if you view a part of your life as unacceptable. I counsel families torn apart by feuds, by squabbles over inheritances and by religious differences. Marrying the 'wrong' person has caused some families to never join together again. How can this be? Even if you and I disagree on every topic, we should still be able to dine together, work together, worship together and even live together. We cannot continue to be broken, or break off our relationships with others, let alone alienate ourselves. As President Clinton spoke to the nation in 1998, "The children of this country can learn in a profound way that integrity is important and selfishness is wrong, but God can change us and make us strong at the broken places."

These fractured relationships can be healed. To have a healthy society and optimal health at a personal level, this healing of families and relationships must happen. But for many, it is a struggle that seems irreconcilable because greater importance has been placed on following a rule or tradition, instead of loving those you birthed or those who birthed you. In your public life, society requires you to embrace all forms of diversity – avoiding all forms of discrimination against race, color, ethnicity, religion, politics and sexual orientation. This rule creates the possibility for a population of diversity to live together. But true diversity begins with a population of one.

You will never live in a world that is free of all prejudice until you embrace the diversity in your own mind and heart. To fall in love with your life and your habit patterns means to become receptive to all the diversity within you. Becoming a creature of charm is to be one who is charmed by your own life and the lives of all whom you meet.

Recently a potential new patient, Ellen, called my office. As is customary, we spoke for 10-15 minutes to get to know each other and determine whether we should work together on her health issues. She was a factory worker who claimed to suffer from post-traumatic stress disorder and depression for the last ten years. Her problems began from stress at work and her list of ailments continued to grow each year – carpal tunnel syndrome, fibromyalgia, stress dermatitis, high blood pressure and a multitude of inflammatory diseases throughout her body. Furthermore, she is seeking legal actions against her employer. Her level of anger and blame was at an all-time high. After listing her medications, she concluded by asking me if I could help her.

On initial telephone interviews, I never really know what is going to happen. With this ambiguity, I answered her in this manner, "Ellen, I do a lot of lecturing at seminars these days. One of the most common questions I ask my audiences that have come to learn about the happiness revolution is: 'Do you want to be right or do you want to be happy?'

"For you, I would modify this question to be: 'Do you want to be right or do you want to get well?'" I went on to explain that revenge is like drinking poison and hoping that the other person will also get sick. "You will have to become a creature of charm if you want to work with me." At that point, she interrupted me to confess that she had never been charming. Her tone of voice told me that she was curious and wanted to know more. I plowed ahead. "I am not asking you to be passive about the policies at your place of work. If something needs to be corrected, then do that, but do not continue to poison yourself with toxic feelings of rage and blame. It will never help you and it will never heal you.

"Are you willing to explore ways to accept all that has happened in your life? At home and at work? Your fault, their fault or nobody's fault? Could you do that? Any and every therapy works better if your mood is charming and kind.

"Diversity is a major buzz word today, but it really means accepting all the diversities and distractions in your life. If you still hate a memory or hide a habit, your level of self-acceptance still needs some polish. You can reduce your pain and heal your body much more easily if a truce has been called on the battlefield within you. Sustainable peace deep within is essential before there can ever be peace in your body and peace in your life – then you will be a creature of charm."

With those words our conversation was drawing to a close. Ellen had become thoughtful and very honest about her emotional life and expectations of her doctors. I asked her to think about our discussion and call me back in 10 days so that we could decide whether we should work together on her ailments. Embracing the diversity of the world begins at home with a population of one. This embrace is love in action. It is a sign of the new times ahead. It is the sign of a new revolution.

THE REVOLUTION HAS BEGUN

We live in a new era. A time that challenges and emboldens our very core. The baby-boomers of the 1950s are aging and seeking their own version of immortality. The number of single adults living alone is higher than ever recorded in human history. Herbal and dietary therapies are now widely accepted and sought after. Longevity and sustainability have become the mantras at the supermarket. The happiness revolution has begun.

I hope these many chapters have offered you new tools and new understandings of how you can find happiness now and in the days to come. We are entering an era of great consequence. Forty years ago

President Kennedy warned us that we have the power to make this the best generation in the history of mankind, or the last. Did Kennedy know that we were about to exceed nature's tolerance for our behavior? Born from our untethered desires to have it all, our lust for acquisition grew and grew. From houses to cars, iPods to televisions, we wanted our own; we did not want to share rides on city buses or live with our relatives. Our desire was never cultivated or disciplined. We wanted what we wanted. None of us knew that the emotional and environmental cost of our demands would be exorbitant and potentially catastrophic. Only transformation at a personal level can begin to stem the tide of this unchecked consumerism.

Having watched and assisted many people in their own self-transformation process, I have seen similar patterns arise spontaneously in their efforts. The following traits and behaviors happen without effort when people consciously choose love as the answer. Happy people do not harm themselves or others. Regardless of their personal past, there dawns a

> *To hear the voice of your conscience is to hear the song of our planet.*

new day when they become firmly established in an eternal union with their conscience. This inner reformation flows outward in every aspect of their life. An awakened mind is a happy mind.

Awakened minds hold themselves to a higher standard. Not only do they do that which is hard, they live in a manner which extols a virtue that cannot be suppressed. There is a light, a brilliance in them that all can see and enjoin. Self-transformation at an individual level eventually births a sense of global unity that will face and defeat all formidable attempts to disrupt nature in its most glorious and most subtle forms.

There is nobility in this call, and there will be sacrifice in this action, as we dedicate a portion of our time and resources to living in greater conformity to the laws of nature. We will continue to raise the bar, until that which we cannot live without -- the oceans and forests, homes and factories, rivers and plants -- have been restored to their rightful place. And you and I must live together as one community on one planet.

To hear the voice of your conscience is to hear the song of our planet. We will surrender that which has never served us well and we will gain that which brings longevity and sustainability to our children and grandchildren. This global movement begins by extending kindness to yourself and those around you. A mass of angry marchers cannot take us where we need to go. You must leave your family, but not your family of parents and children. You must leave your family of desires and doubts, which obstructs your view of the world and all living beings.

> *The happiness revolution will occur as spontaneous bands of individuals, families and communities choose kindness and sustainability over fads and fears.*

It is time for us to re-evaluate the value and the consequences of our lifestyles. Self-discipline and self-regulation cannot be imposed from the outside. Discipline is the internal process of evaluation and renewal of self-effort. To be a disciple of goodness means to discipline one's self for a higher good, a higher reward. The happiness revolution will occur as spontaneous bands of individuals, families and communities choose kindness and sustainability over fads and fears.

CONCLUSION

To join the happiness revolution, gather your courage to dismantle unhealthy beliefs and thought patterns that will never support your goal of peace and happiness. Sharpen your mind and learn to reject those opinions that keep you scared or lonely. The more you hear and heed the voice of your own heart, the easier it will be to let the tedium and misery from the past fall from your attention.

This is not the time to become passive. You will need to have a strong and cultured ego. Rather than attempting to kill your ego, try expanding your ego to include those around you. Eventually, let your ego expand to include all of us. Train your ego so that you can be confident and do your work. Do not be afraid of people and do not be afraid of your ego -- it is your friend and can become a great ally. Develop self-confidence about your own validity; this will free you from needing outside validation.

Use this book and every resource that you have available to design a holistic model for living that works for you and your family. Let common sense and practicality be the

> *Develop self-confidence about your own validity.*

source of this model. Keep encouraging your mind to close all the doors on potential obstacles. Any fascination with failure and frustration will wear down as the light within you becomes more captivating than the shadows.

In the next phase of growth, we will see good and kind people become generous and focused on service to others. Humanity cannot become inert. Our inner commotion is coming to an end, as the light of this new era has re-kindled the light within us. The spirit of humanity is calling out to all of us to become a light to ourselves. It beckons us to develop trust in ourselves, in our innate abilities, in our kinsmen, in God and in the eternal law that clearly explains the relationship between sowing and reaping. No one out there is the cause of your grace or your misery – you are the sole creator of your happiness.

Longevity is born from vision. A world of hope and happiness inspires enthusiasm and creativity. Why would anyone want to live a long life, if their daily life is unpleasant?   The lifestyle and skill-sets that foster happiness will simultaneously foster health and rejuvenation. As you choose to live a quality life, the quantity of time allotted to you may expand. However, my patients continually teach me that their quality of life and love

> *The lifestyle and skill-sets that foster happiness will simultaneously foster health and rejuvenation.*

is much more precious than the number of years that they live.

Finally, don't assume that this book was written for anyone other than you. For who is more deserving of happiness than you? No one. Finding your purpose has nothing to do with your profession, income level, or social status. When you know yourself, your place in the world and how wonderful you are, then you are starting to fulfill the purpose of your life -- this is where happiness is born.

He who wants to do good, knocks at the gate;
he who loves, finds the gates open.
-- Rabindranath Tagore (1861-1941)

CHAPTER SUMMARY

- We would do well to remember that all the great sages declare that love supersedes everything.
- Awakened minds are held to a higher standard. Not only must we do that which is hard, we must live that which extols a virtue that cannot be suppressed.
- We will surrender that which has never served us well and we will gain that which brings longevity and sustainability to our children and grandchildren. This global movement begins by extending kindness to yourself and those around you.

Acknowledgments

I am forever grateful to everyone who shared their lives and insights with me. Continually my main inspiration to write and teach comes from the potential for greatness and happiness I see in the hearts and lives of my patients, friends and family.

It is the loving guidance of Pandit Rajmani Tigunait, Ph.D. that has allowed me to see solutions to physical and emotional suffering where many said there was none. He encouraged me to re-work Ayurveda into a format that addresses the lifestyle and stresses of today. Thank you, Panditji, for your untiring efforts to teach and guide me in this work.

The love of my family and friends has been overwhelming. No matter how much I travel or sequester myself to type, they are there for me in every way imaginable. I am so happy to have this book dedicated to my mother, Barbara Ann Lewis.

Marc and Astrid Vaccaro constantly reflected on my ideas and the problems our society faces today. They kept reminding me to speak from my heart and share the truth of my experience. Thank you for your unending love and support.

In the writing phase, Todd Wolfenberg, once again, escaped from the world to spend over a year of dictation and rewrites on this book. Jordan Shapiro traveled with me for a month taking dictation on planes and late nights in hotels along my east coast lecture tour and conference schedule. Deven Karvelas edited and reviewed many of the ideas I tried so clearly to convey, while Todd and Dana awaited the birth of their son, Maxx. Deven created the chapter summaries and many of the recipes.

My editors were amazing. Writing is a very solitary profession that makes a writer face himself on paper. It is the editor's job to bring comic relief and clarity when the written words started to blur on the Macintosh. Cathy Dean and Celia Rocks assisted with the beginning stages of this work. PJ Slinger then took charge of pulling this book together with his insightful comments and masterful editing skills. Finally, Elizabeth Place and Lisa Lewis came in for the final edit and transformed this into a great book. Lisa, Elizabeth and PJ have made the editing work an incredible experience of learning and fellowship. Thank you Cathy, Celia, PJ, Elizabeth and Lisa.

I sought special counsel from Luke Ketterhagen (www.hathapower. com), Chad Oler, N.D. and Jon Hinds for their expertise in hatha, nutrition and fitness, respectively. All three I consider leaders in their field and teachers to the masses. Luke continually brings insight and wonder to hatha yoga and teaches advanced training in all the yogic sciences around the country. Dr. Oler lectures around the nation and continues to see patients at the Natural Path Center in Madison, Wisconsin (www.naturalpathhealthcenter.com). Jon Hinds is bringing fitness to corporate America and to people all over the world through his seminars and fitness equipment. You can find Jon at www.jonhinds. com/cnt/ and www.monkeybargym.com. Thank you all.

In searching for better ways to express my thoughts, I dined and debated with David and Betty Holloway. David is a psychiatrist creating new holistic models for mental health care, while Betty continues to use her academic credentials and culinary talent to teach the finest courses in vegetarian cooking. She and Deven Karvelas wrote the recipes in this book. Thank you so much.

Rick Das Goravani spent several hours in tutoring me in some of the finer concepts of time management according to the science of Jyotish. Thank you Rick for your time and encouragement.

Jeff Hiser returned to illustrate this second work for me. His artistic flair for realism and precision is seen in every drawing. Thank you Jeff.

My research team, led by Todd Wolfenberg, included Chelsea Wolfenberg, Jordan Shapiro, and Deven Karvelas. Thank you all for your weekends, evenings, and daylight hours of reading, Googling, and verifying these works. These folks fed me, made the best chai in the world, and challenged me to think bigger than ever before. I feel honored to have such a diligent team that demands something greater than mere excellence from me and from themselves.

Then comes a huge host of supporters, readers, and critics, including Gabe Colton leading the charge for the first critical reading of this text, with the assistance of many, including Bob Mattingly, Jackie Dobrinska, Bernie Rosen, Tammy Mehlberg, Don Ashbaugh, Jeff Abella, Josh Wolfenberg, Shanon Samuson, Travis Head, Matt and Briana Douzart, Michael Daly of Dublin, Susan Crofton, Varuna Singh, Amala and Andy Heeter, Carrie Demers MD, Donna and Kay Eckstein, Michael Maloney, Ray Purdy MD, Karen Host, Doug Frazer, Whitney Vallier, David Cadwallader, Terri Oswald-Plonske, MD, Tiffany Hacker, Kendall Inman, Kelly Ullmer, Nicholas Karvelas, David and Betty Holloway, Luke and Kourtney Ketterhagen, Linda Orton, Bob and Donna Abella, Marc and Astrid Vacarro, Terri Wickman, Ed Mills, Lisa Renard, Jon Hinds and Jessica Rucker, Jane and Dana Marski, and Danielle Ruffalo. The list continues with John and Jan Wolfenberg, Monica and Josiah Groth, Lisa Lewis, Kevin Loecher, Sally Lewis, J'Gai and Faraji Starks, Jeff Starks and my mother, Barbara Lewis. Your generosity came from every direction and in every form. And I needed it all.

The thoughtful design elements of the cover and interior pages were made possible from the incredibly creative team led by Allen D'Angelo and Kimberly Leonard at Bookcovers.com. Thank you for this beautiful look and your huge support in marketing this epistle.

A special thank you to all of the volunteers, administrators, staff, and students at the Alive and Healthy Institute and at the Blue Sky Educational Foundation.

And to Karen, thank you for your love and support. We traveled well together.

Blair Lewis

"No medicine will cure what happiness will not."

About the Author

Blair Lewis, PA, is a licensed physician assistant, specializing in the use of homeopathy, Ayurveda, nutrition, and the yogic sciences to prevent and resolve chronic ailments.

Blair is the author of *Happiness: The Real Medicine and How It Works* and a co-author of *Homeopathic Remedies for Health Professionals and Laypeople*. He has also written several e-books, along with a host of articles and interviews on holistic health. In 1985, he co-founded the Blue Sky Educational Foundation, a nonprofit organization teaching the leading innovations of massage and holistic health.

For over 20 years Blair has been actively teaching and consulting with patients and audiences world-wide. Today, Blair continues his study of yoga science, tantra and ayurveda under the guidance of Pandit Tigunait and the tradition of the Himalayan Institute.

Blair is the creator and spiritual director of the Alive and Healthy Institute. Since 2002, the Alive and Healthy Institute has sought to improve the lives of all people worldwide by building a bridge between science and spirituality. The Foundation's main outreach to the global community is accomplished through lectures and seminars, humanitarian outreach projects, the distribution of free e-zines (newsletters) and free e-books on science and spirituality. The Alive and Healthy Institute is a Sacred Link Affiliate of the Himalayan Institute and is located on the internet at: www.AliveandHealthy.com.

An enthusiastic teacher and author, Blair offers seminars and retreats on Ayurvedic rejuvenation and yoga science. He attended both the National Center for Homeopathy (1983) and the International Foundation for Homeopathy (1985). A graduate of Indiana University and the Physician Assistant Program at Lake Erie College and the Cleveland Clinic Foundation, he has also studied in Europe, Greece, and India. You can reach Blair for seminars and private consultations at:

www.AliveandHealthy.com
and
www.BlairLewis.com

"When you know yourself, your place in the world and how wonderful you are, then you are starting to fulfill the purpose of your life."
— Blair Lewis

APPENDIX A
Chapter Summaries

CHAPTER 1: STURDY BODY AND STABLE MIND

"Without fear and possessiveness, stress cannot exist."

Summary

- Happiness is your true nature. When you regain the stability of your mind and the sturdiness of your body, then health and happiness will return in full force.
- What you store in your mind will shape your experience of life.
- Your buddhi (conscience) is the guard at the gate into your mind. It can help you choose what you allow in and what you discard.

Action Items

- Practice trying to distinguish between the thoughts presented by your buddhi and the thoughts presented by your ego.
- Practice extracting the most useful and positive wisdom from every life experience, regardless of whether the experience itself was pleasant or unpleasant.

"Happiness has not forsaken you, rather you have forsaken it."

CHAPTER 2: KNOW YOURSELF
DETERMINING YOUR AYURVEDIC CONSTITUTION

"Throughout human history, the concept of self-understanding has been fundamental to virtually every culture and religion."

Summary

- To know which path will take you to happiness, you must first know who you are, what you are and what resources you have available.

- Understanding the three Ayurvedic constitutions will provide you with a foundation from which you can go on to understand yourself at deeper levels.

- When you make your choices in life with respect to your knowledge of yourself and your constitution, you will be less likely to suffer from imbalances in any area of life.

Action Items

- Take the "Ayurvedic Quiz" to find out your constitution.

- Make a list of activities you engage in or foods or beverages you consume that may not be helpful for your constitution.

"To know which path to take, you must first know who you are, what you are and what resources you have available."

Chapter 3: Living with Purpose

*"You may not be living the life you want,
but you can enjoy living the life you have."*

The Five Principles of Living With Purpose

Principle One: Do No Harm (most important)
Summary
- In the practice of non-violence, the most important component and essential starting point is non-violence toward yourself. Never condemn, criticize or punish yourself.

Action Item
- Practice rewarding yourself and actively engaging in not criticizing yourself.

Principle Two: Truthfulness
Summary
- Truthfulness is valuable, but only so long as it is not violent to ourselves or to others. Truthfulness must be skillfully practiced along with the principle of non-violence, which always comes first.

Action Item:
- Before speaking or acting, think beyond your truthfulness and consider whether or not you are also being loving and compassionate.

Principle Three: Abstain From All Forms of Theft
Summary
- The principle of abstaining from theft is attained naturally when one realizes that "the possessions of others – physical

and non-physical -- can neither fulfill nor threaten your happiness."

Action Item

- Examine your life for things which are not yours, but which you cling to or desire nonetheless. Acknowledge that they do not belong to you and let go of your attachment to them.

Principle Four: Moving Through the World with a Unified Mind

Summary

- Learning to control your senses and gently guiding them to engage in constructive and helpful activities will allow you to begin obtaining freedom from the intensity of sensory cravings. In their place, you will begin to experience your inward dwelling joy.

Action Item

- In order to practice the concept of "do not suppress and do not indulge," the next time you desire something which is not helpful for you, say to yourself: "That's all right for my mind to desire that object, but I have control over my body and I will not go and get that object for my mind."

Principle Five: Freedom from Possessiveness

Summary

- Becoming dependent upon either physical objects in the world or any identity that you have constructed for yourself will not improve your ability to find happiness, it will limit it.

Action Item

- Contemplate what you consider to be your identity and your possessions, and then contemplate what would be left if you had none of those objects or ideas.

Five Daily Observances for Living with Purpose

Cleanliness and Purity
Summary
- When you recognize your own inner purity, you will begin to make decisions in life that support and maintain that purity in an internal and external sense.

Action Item
- Pick something simple (make a small healthy change in your diet, try a pranayama exercise, clean a part of your living space that is typically cluttered, etc...) to add a little cleanliness to your life. Observe the effect it has on you.

Contentment
Summary
- Contentment requires you to actively choose to be content – regardless of your circumstances.

Action Item
- Practice being content in a situation in which you would not normally feel content.

Self-Effort
Summary
- Even a small amount of self-effort, when sincere and in the right direction, will always yield results and can inspire you to make greater efforts to achieve greater results.

Action Item
- Choose a simple point of guidance from this book and make an effort to practice it in your life, and observe the results.

Self-Study

Summary

- Self-study is your opportunity to take something home from the classroom of life experiences. Examine your experiences in life in combination with guidance from books, teachers and therapists to gain insights and guidance to help you toward your goals.

Action Item

- Set aside a practical, realistic amount of quiet time for regular self-study.

Spiritual Clarity – The End of Selfishness

Summary

- At this highest point of self-realization, you have recognized the equalities of all people, and that the entire field of life, in all of its forms, constitutes a single being.

Action Item

- In order to evolve beyond personal prejudices, practice observing the similarities between you and people whom you previously thought of as different from you.

_"The only way we can harm ourselves is to
ignore the voice of our conscience."_

Chapter 4: The Happiness Diet

"You can learn to eat simply so that others can simply eat."

Summary

A few basic principles on how and what you eat will guide you toward the quality of life you seek.

- Foods have a powerful impact on your moods and emotions. If you keep eating the same way, you will keep feeling the same way.
- Foods determine your health status, longevity and the appearance of your body. Most diseases and deaths can be attributed to the patient's diet. Likewise, longevity and happiness can be attributed to the diet.
- Foods can feed you or feed many. Today we live in a global community and our harvest belongs to everyone. Your diet can support the feeding of millions or the feeding of the fortunate few.

To live a healthier lifestyle, follow these simple dietary ideas.

- Reduce and consider removing fast food, junk food, and overly processed foods from your diet. Home-cooked meals will make it easy for you to avoid foods with added salt or sugar, refined sugars and refined grains.
- Limit dairy and meat consumption (especially ice cream and aged cheese).
- Add fruits and vegetables.
- Add whole grains.
- Switch to healthy oils.
- Replace soda, alcohol, coffee and sweetened juices with water.

- Enjoy your meal in a calm peaceful environment. Take time to chew your food thoroughly. Try to eat at regular times throughout the week.

"Your garden and your shopping cart can replace your psychologist and your internist and help to solve global starvation."

Chapter 5: Hatha Yoga

"Exercise will improve your overall health,
state of mind and quality of life."

Summary

- In everyday life, when we perform practical actions such as walking, lifting, running, pushing and jumping, we do not use our muscle groups in isolation.

- Whatever is the first point of resistance in your exercise, be it your feet or hands or head, from that point on, you have to be stabilized.

- The greater stability you have at each joint the less likelihood you have of injury.

- Engage your muscles from the inside out, learn how they feel. Your tone, strength and function will improve over time as you activate, contract or expand your body. Remember, engagement usually begins in the hands and the feet. But more importantly, please remember that freedom of movement is the ultimate goal.

- In hatha yoga there is a systematic series of postures and stretches that help strengthen and rebalance the body.

- The complete practice of hatha always includes breath awareness and pranayama. These ancient exercises have a profound ability to balance, cleanse, and rejuvenate the physical and energetic body.

- Turn your attention inward. Stay aware of your breath. Relax and breathe serenely in every posture. Your hatha practice is the most comprehensive way to explore and heal yourself.

"The most important thing to remember about exercise
is that any amount is better than none."

CHAPTER 6: HOMEOPATHY: THE ENERGY MEDICINE

"It is the simplicity, safety, and quality of homeopathy that makes it so appealing today."

Summary

- Homeopathy often helps people overcome physical and psychological problems when other therapies have failed and the problem seems impossible to overcome.
- Homeopathic medicines have the unique ability to help you get through difficult situations. Sometimes, when you get stuck in a bout of sadness and grief, homeopathy can help release pent-up feelings that you have suppressed and bring you back to a state of happiness.
- In an age when antibiotics are becoming ineffective and diseases are more easily transmitted, homeopathy offers great hope for the future.

"Homeopathic medicine is the most powerful, fast-acting, and completely safe therapy in the world."

Chapter 7: Sleep, Rest and Relaxation

Summary

- Rest and relaxation exercises are cleansing techniques. Rest removes dullness and inertia while relaxation removes restlessness and anxiety.

- Rest and relaxation are important prerequisites to good sleep. If you go to sleep anxious and restless, your quality of sleep will suffer.

Action Items

- Practice one full round of alternate nostril breathing each day for 11 days and observe the effect.

- Practice the 61-point relaxation exercise daily until you can complete the exercise regularly without falling asleep.

CHAPTER 8: YOGA NIDRA: THE SCIENCE OF YOGIC SLEEP

"Rest and relaxation are cleansing techniques that can have a profound impact on your life and your relationships."

Summary

- Sleep doesn't always provide good rest. It is quite possible to sleep eight hours and still be tired if the sleep was of poor quality. Therefore it is important to learn to sleep properly.

- What you eat, watch, listen to, think about and do in the hours before sleeping will affect the quality of your sleep dramatically.

- Through the science of yoga and the practice of yoga nidra, it is possible to gain deep rest in a short period of time.

Action Items

- Take note of your behaviors in the four or five hours before sleeping, and use the information presented in this chapter, along with the "checklist for a rest-less night" to determine which of those behaviors are helpful and which are unhelpful.

- Begin either the prerequisite practices for yoga nidra or the actual practice of yoga nidra as described in this chapter.

"To be happy and healthy, you have to stop being a victim to your dietary habits, your breathing patterns and your sleeping patterns."

Chapter 9: Creating More Space for Happiness

If you learn how to have more space in your day, it will feel like you have more time.

Summary

- You can't change time, but you can change your experience of time by creating more space, flexibility and vitality in your body through the practice of hatha yoga and pranayama.

- Controlling your breath is the quickest way to control your mind. Your breathing patterns have great influence over your experience of life.

Action Items

- Set aside a practical amount of time everyday for yourself to stretch and work with your breath using the alternate nostril breathing technique, described in Chapter 7, and hatha yoga exercises from Chapter 5 of this book.

- Try the counting exercise explained in this chapter for 11 days.

- Create a practical but consistent schedule to experiment with the Advanced Relaxation exercise outlined in chapter seven.

"Hatha yoga and pranayama can expand your capacity by helping you stretch and expand yourself."

Chapter 10: Filling Your Day with Happiness

"In the pursuit of happiness, time management is absolutely essential."

Summary
- You can change the influence of your past experiences by changing your perception of the past.
- There are natural rhythms to time and to our experience of life. If you understand and cooperate with these rhythms, your life will flow smoother and you will struggle less.
- Thinking about and planning your life in 25-year blocks of time will help you lead a life that will be fulfilling to you and allow you to work toward uncovering the highest joy in life.

Action Items
- Write down the things from your past which you are still actively involved in trying to change or simply never let go of. Consider the freedom that you would gain by letting go of these experiences.
- Regardless of your actual age, decide which of the four phases of life discussed in this chapter you are in right now. Then contemplate how you would like your life to be in the remaining phases and plan out what you need to do to make those visions a reality.
- Review the times of the day when each Ayurvedic constitution is dominant, and which activities are most favorable during these times. Take note of how much of your life fits into this pattern and how much is in conflict with it. Experiment with changing those conflicting activities and notice the results.

"The only escape from the past is to live in the present – a present that remains uncontaminated by the past."

Chapter 11: A Life of Balance and Harmony

"Contemplation hones and refines your ability to listen to your conscience."

Summary

- Contemplation helps you endow your life with clarity and purpose. It will ensure that you gain wisdom and guidance from your life experiences and move forward in a positive direction rather than repeating aimless cycles of events.

- Contemplation is the art of skillfully guiding your internal dialogue in a manner that helps you reflect on who you are, what you are doing, why you are doing it, how you will do it and what you have learned from your past experiences.

- The unconscious mind needs to be stirred by some stimulus from the conscious mind in order to be activated. Contemplation, with full determination, on positive attributes and ideas will prevent unhelpful tendencies from arising in your mind.

Action Items

- If you worship any particular god or concept of divinity, write down the positive attributes your concept of god has and do your best to imitate these.

- Choose five phrases, quotes, or helpful sayings from this book, or elsewhere, that you feel could help to guide your decisions and reactions on a daily basis.

"The power of strong determination is greater than the urges of the subconscious mind."

CHAPTER 12: ACQUIRING A JOYFUL MIND

*"Meditation will allow you to observe firsthand the nature
of your mind and the nature of your self."*

Summary

- The practice of meditation will allow you to observe firsthand the nature of your mind and the nature of your self (your conscience) and discover that there is a sharp difference between these two.
- The literal meaning of meditation is the process of paying attention. What you pay attention to, or the object of your meditation, will determine the results you experience. Using a mantra as an object of meditation will help prevent you from wasting your time by meditating on discomfort in your body or emotions that you may be feeling.
- When meditating, thoughts will arise. It is important to let these thoughts come and go without becoming disturbed by them. It is better to focus on increasing your awareness of your mantra than to try to suppress other thoughts.

Action Items

- Keep a journal of your private thoughts and feelings, and see whether this practice provides you with any insights or clarifications in your life.
- Choose a regular activity that you engage in now, that is either unhelpful or unnecessary in your life, and replace it with time for learning to meditate.
- Practice meditation on the *Soham* mantra as described in this chapter and keep a journal of your experience.

*"Depending upon the relationship you have with your mind, your
moments of solitude will either be pleasant or unpleasant."*

Chapter 13: Discovering Our Sacred Link

"It is said that when the student is ready, the teacher will appear."

Summary

- Before you can master your emotions, you must feel like a master. When you perform your actions like a slave, then all you are doing is working. But when you perform your actions like a master, then there is a graciousness and a selflessness that greases your actions.

- To build a firm foundation of peace within you, all levels of your life have to come into balance. That is why it takes many years for most of us to achieve that solid inner core and outer core of stability in our life.

- Good intentions are not enough. Good intentions should be put into action. We cannot force others to change, but we can change ourselves and become an example to the world.

"Every skilled master of every trade was once an apprentice, and every teacher once a student".

CHAPTER 14: LOVE AND LONGEVITY

"Keep encouraging your mind to close all the doors of potential obstacles."

Summary

- We would do well to remember that all the great sages declare that love supersedes everything.

- Awakened minds are held to a higher standard. Not only must we do that which is hard, we must live that which extols a virtue that cannot be suppressed.

- We will surrender that which has never served us well and we will gain that which brings longevity and sustainability to our children and grandchildren. This global movement begins by extending kindness to yourself and those around you.

"When you know yourself, your place in the world and how wonderful you are, then you are starting to fulfill the purpose of your life."

APPENDIX B

To assist your ability to hear the voice of your conscience, as discusssed in Chapter 11, I have included this special contemplation practice. If you read and consider this message once a day for the next 11 days, I am confident that it will help you. Please take a moment and review Chaper 11.

There is no other
by Blair Lewis
August 3, 2006

Until you hear my voice, there is no other voice worth hearing.

Until you heed my voice, there is no other worth heeding.

You may need tragedy to interrupt all your distractions in order to find me. However, you need not seek out such drama, simply quiet your restless body and breath. This will soothe your mind and soon I will appear.

On a quiet morning, sit still. Compare these two voices as you recite the following in the privacy of your mind: "I am here, I need nothing." And, "I want this, I fear that!" Repeat it over and over until you can hear the difference.

Until you can hear me, there is no one else to listen to.

Many people will come and go in your life. They always have and they always will. But I am your one faithful companion. I am that which brings insight, clarity, laughter and love to every moment.

You may offend them or you may serve them, but until you serve me, you are only a victim or puppet of others. I am the only way. Have no other Gods before me, including television, the suggestions and opinions of others, memory, desire, fear, intellect or hatred. If there is a larger picture, a God of the heavens, a prince or princess of peace, you will not find them or see them, until you know me. It is through me that all is known and all is seen.

Until you hear my voice, the voices of others will please you, confuse you and frighten you. There is no way you can ever organize and assimilate the events of this world until you bond with me.

I am known by many names, but in truth I am most easily known by your name. When your beloved calls out your name, your lover is not calling out to your mind, but rather to you. Not the memories, not the histories, not the recent past or the fantasies of the future, but here and now, your beloved wants you. And I am that.

I am your conscience. When you see me as your true identity and no longer mistake yourself for your personal past, your desires, or your errors, then you will forsake all these trappings and join me. Then you will be at peace.

Everyone wants you. Everyone uses you for their own needs. In return, you try to use them to satisfy your wants and desires. It works a lot of the time, but the achievements are short-lived. They claim to love you and want to be with you forever. But, someday all of them will leave. The only one who will always be with you is me.

Why keep trying to please them, find them, or use them? It is a hoax that it will help you.

Once you recognize me, enjoin with me, merge into me, then the world is your toy and everything becomes a possibility. No longer will fear hold you back or lust drive you into a corner. Your ability to love others becomes unlimited and life becomes grand.

Once you know me, once you are me, then all that ever was and ever will be, is yours.

You only need to pause and consider the possibility of my existence. I am the love you seek.

I leave you with these comments:

I Am The Great Sun

I am the great Sun, but you do not see me.
I am your Husband, but you turn away.
I am the Captive, but you do not free me.
I am the Captain you will not obey.
I am the Truth, but you will not believe me.
I am the City, where you will not stay.
I am your Wife, your Child, but you will leave me.
I am that God, to whom you will not pray.
I am your Counsel, but you do not hear me.
I am the Lover, whom you will betray.
I am the Victor, but you do not cheer me.
I am the Holy Dove, whom you will slay.
I am your Life, but if you will not name me,
Seal up your soul with tears and never blame me.

Charles Causley, Norman Crucifix, 1632.

I am waiting – ever calling, ever loving, ever waiting.

Because there is no other.

.

APPENDIX C
Recipes for Happiness

The following is a sampling of recipes to nourish you and your family. Use the recipes as an experimental base as you search for a diet that you find delicious and helpful in your efforts to become established in happiness. A good meal should be pleasing to your senses and calming to your mind.

I have included some information about ghee, a few spices and some important foods before delving into the actual recipes. Spices have the ability to help your food be more digestible and to enhance the flavor of the food. Ghee is the supreme cooking oil and merits a wholesome introduction.

Please feel welcome to contribute recipes to this effort. I would love to share your recipes online with all of the families, book clubs and organizations reading this book. You can send them to "Recipes@AliveandHealthy.com."

Thank you very much for your thoughtful attention and curiosity.

Blair Lewis

Extras:

GHEE — CLARIFIED BUTTER

Cooking with Ghee

Ghee is the perfect cooking oil. Since all of the water and milk solids are removed from butter in the process of making ghee, ghee will not burn while cooking. It is a very stable oil, even at high cooking temperatures. Unlike many vegetable oil alternatives, it is not prone to forming free radicals, which lead to tissue damage, premature aging and abnormal behavior of cells in a carcinogenic manner. It contains no trans-fatty acids, which have been linked to higher rates of cancer and heart disease. In addition to all of this, it adds a wonderful flavor and aroma to your cooking.

Like all oils, ghee should be used in moderation.

Ayurveda and Ghee

Ghee has three important properties in Ayurvedic medicine. It is said to cure Vatic disturbances, diminish or cool the fire of Pitta and supply and replenish Kapha. These qualities make it a uniquely perfect food to consume when practicing intense forms of pranayama, during which Vatic disturbances can be created, excessive heat is generated and the body mass might become detrimentally reduced.

Ayurveda teaches that ghee has a special capacity for picking up the medicinal effects of seasonings and herbs and carrying them into the body. For this reason, many Ayurvedic herbs are prepared in a ghee base.

Butyric Acid

The actions of butyric acid (a short-chain fatty acid produced in the rumen of the cow from fermented vegetation) seems to be responsible for many of the health benefits provided by ghee. Butyric acid can be obtained in the diet either through butterfat or through dietary fiber, which produces butyric acid when it is fermented in the colon. Butyric acid is helpful for the overall health and maintenance of the cells in the lining of the colon. In addition to this it provides antiviral properties by increasing the level of a molecule called interferon.[15] It also possesses anti-cancer properties and has been shown to inhibit and even reverse malignant growth.[16] It may be particularly helpful in preventing colon cancer. Part of this may be due to the fact that Butyric acid reduces colonic pH and inhibits secondary bile acids, which may be carcinogenic.[17] Ayurveda prizes ghee as a treatment for Vatic disturbances. Since Ayurveda also views the large intestines as the abode of Vata, it makes sense that ghee would improve intestinal health.

ONIONS

The onion is a wonderful addition to many common soups, sandwiches, and salads. Onions add flavor, richness and energy to many meals. Onions stimulate the immune system and have an overall warming effect on the body. A moderate amount of the pungent taste of onions stimulates salivation and the digestive fire, destroys pathogens and dries out Kapha, making it good for use in preventing respiratory diseases.

Consumption of too many onions can aggravate Pitta, causing headaches and inflammation. Pittas should generally avoid raw onions. Vatas can handle cooked onions and small amounts of raw onions in their diet. Kaphas are able to withstand more liberal amounts of both raw and cooked onions, though cooked onions are still preferred. However, for acute illnesses and colds, both raw and cooked onions have tremendous merit in their healing properties.

GARLIC

Garlic is one of the most powerful and helpful herbs both in cooking and in medicine. Garlic is ubiquitous in Italian and Greek cook-

ing as well as in many other cuisines from around the world. Current
Western research on garlic states that the medicinal effects of garlic
are most powerful if garlic is taken raw, immediately after crushing
the clove.

According to Ayurveda, garlic is a stimulating, warming food. The
ability of garlic to increase Pitta makes it useful in Kaphic disorders,
such as congestion, depression, obesity, and sluggishness. For excessive mucus, raw or cooked garlic can be used. As a food spice, garlic
is most effective in oil, so sautéed garlic is considered the best method
of use.

GINGER

Ginger is a root vegetable that is used commonly in Asian cooking. In Ayurveda, ginger is one of the most cleansing spices. It is
particularly useful as a digestive aid and for calming nausea. The
anti-inflammatory properties of ginger are also helpful in treating the
pain and inflammation associated with osteo- and rheumatoid arthritis. Boiled in water, and taken with lemon and honey as a beverage,
ginger tea can be helpful in easing sore throats, coughs, colds, and
other respiratory disorders. Ginger can be obtained as a fresh root or
as a powder. Both forms of ginger are effective, however, fresh ginger
root is preferred.

TURMERIC

Turmeric is a bright-yellow root spice used in Indian cooking. Recently, research has validated the healing and anti-inflammatory aspects of turmeric, which have long been recognized in ancient healing
traditions. In Ayurveda it is famous as a tonic for pain. Turmeric
can be ingested or made into a paste or oil and applied externally for
painful joints and blemishes; however, due to the staining nature of
turmeric, people rarely use it today. Aside from its widespread health

benefits, turmeric is a great tasting spice to include in your cooking. Served in your food, turmeric will provide antioxidants and aid in digestion. This spice has warming qualities, but is not hot like cayenne or other peppers.

Be careful handling turmeric, as it will stain anything it touches bright yellow. I have many wooden spoons, plastic containers, and articles of clothing that have been stained by this otherwise wonderful spice.

CUMIN

Cumin is a popular spice in Mexican cooking and also has medicinal qualities. Cumin reduces gas and is helpful for digestive disorders. Cumin can be used as an antidote to overeating and heavy meals, soothing distention and abdominal pain and helping to digest bread. In Ayurveda, dry roasted cumin seeds are ground up and blended with plain yogurt. One tablespoon of roasted, ground cumin in one cup of yogurt is a great aid to digestion for adults. Cumin is also known for its diuretic effects and its helpfulness with nausea and morning sickness.

CORIANDER

Coriander is probably one of the first spices used by mankind, having been known as early as 5000 BC. Sanskrit writings dating from about 1500 BC also spoke of it. Coriander seed comes from the cilantro plant. Just as cilantro is often put in salsa and Mexican dishes to cool off and balance the spiciness, coriander seed also has cooling properties. In addition, coriander is commonly used in lentil and other bean dishes, as it counteracts the tendency for them to cause Vatic imbalances in the form of flatulence. Coriander is also used as a digestive stimulant, and aids in the digestion of cruciferous vegetables.

DEEP COLORED BERRIES

Deep colored berries, such as blackberries, cranberries, raspberries, and blueberries are generally considered to be tridoshic, helping Vatas, Pittas and Kaphas. This is because berries have sweet, light, and cooling qualities. Vatas benefit from the sweet taste of berries, Kaphas benefit from the lightness of most berries, and Pittas are aided by the cooling properties of berries. These wonderful gifts of nature make a delicious and healthy snack loaded with healthy nutrients and antioxidants.

LEAFY GREENS

Leafy green vegetables like spinach, romaine lettuce, kale and collard greens are a great source of many vitamins, minerals, enzymes and antioxidants. The darker green leafy vegetables provide the most benefit. Colorless vegetables, like iceberg lettuce, have less benefit and nutritional value. As a general rule of thumb, the greener the plant, the more nutrients you will get from it. Though some leafy greens have salty, sweet, pungent, and/or sour tastes, the most prevalent taste of most greens is bitter. Their enzymes, vitamins (A, C, E, and K), and minerals (iron, calcium, magnesium) make them highly recommended by all traditions of healing. Leafy greens can be either tender and lightly flavored, or hardy and strong flavored.

The method of the preparation of greens determines their nutritional value. Chopping and cooking leafy greens before consumption helps increase their digestibility. Cooking leafy greens is usually either done by steaming, sautéing in ghee, or cooking with a dal, soup, or grain. Tender leafy greens take only a few minutes to cook down, while the more hardy varieties can take up to 20 minutes. Some greens such as spinach and lettuce are tender enough to be eaten raw in salads. Vatas and Pittas should avoid eating too many hardy greens, while favoring tender greens cooked with proper spices.

Kaphas can consume tender and hardy varieties of leafy greens, but they should still be cooked and spiced appropriately for their constitution.

Breakfasts

Scrambled Tofu
(serves 3-4)

1 small onion chopped
1 lb. block of firm tofu (squish with hands in a mixing bowl, don't leave any large chunks)
6 cloves crushed garlic
½ cup frozen peas
2 chopped tomatoes
1 T brown mustard seeds
2 t turmeric
1 t cumin
1 t ginger powder
1 t coriander
1/8 t black pepper
3 T ghee (clarified butter)
½ cup water
Salt to taste

Step one: Sauté the onion in the ghee on medium heat until translucent. Add all spices; then after stirring for about 30 seconds, add the ½ cup of water.

Step two: Stir in the tofu and the garlic so that the spices mix well with the tofu.

Step three: Add the frozen peas and tomatoes. Cook for five to ten minutes until peas are soft and warm. Add water if it starts to stick while cooking. Salt to taste.

Bran Muffins
(Makes 18-20 muffins)

Dry ingredients
3 cups whole wheat pastry flour
1 cup unbleached flour
1½ T baking soda
½ T salt

Wet ingredients
2 cups wheat bran
½ cup boiling water
1½ cups maple syrup
¾ cup ghee (clarified butter)
3 cups buttermilk
¾ cup raisins
½ cup eggs

Step one: Preheat oven to 350 degrees.

Step two: Mix together and set aside the dry ingredients.

Step three: Toss together the bran and hot water. Add the other wet ingredients, then stir in the dry ingredients.

Step four: Bake in oiled and flour dusted muffin tins for 30-40 minutes.

Note: Batter will keep for up to 3-5 days if refrigerated. Store with plastic wrap directly on the surface of the batter.

Whole Wheat Pancakes
(Serves 3-4)

Dry ingredients
2 cups whole wheat pastry flour
1 T brown sugar
½ t cinnamon
4 t baking powder
1 t salt

Wet ingredients
2 cups milk
¾ cup water
½ cup apple sauce
2 T ghee (clarified butter)
1 t vanilla

Step one: Sift the dry ingredients together.

Step two: Mix the wet ingredients together, then pour into the dry mixture while stirring with a whisk.

Step three: Cook on an oiled frying pan or griddle. Flip the pancakes when little bubbles begin to form across the uncooked side of the pancake. Both sides of the pancake should be golden brown when done. If the center is not cooking well enough, try a lower heat.

Lunches

Pesto Pasta
(serves 3-4)

1 chopped onion
8 sliced mushrooms
4-6 cloves of crushed garlic
6 oz. fresh basil leaves
½ cup pine nuts
1/3 cup olive oil (goes in blender)
2 T olive oil (for sautéing in frying pan)
1 T lemon juice
1/3 cup water
2-3 chopped tomatoes
2 T Italian seasoning
1 t salt
1 box of spaghetti or the pasta of your choice

Step one: Sauté the onion on medium heat in 2 tablespoons of olive oil until translucent. Then add the sliced mushrooms, garlic and Italian seasoning. Continue to sauté until mushrooms are well cooked (about 10 minutes).

Step two: Toast the pine nuts for 5-7 minutes at 350 degrees or until golden brown.

Step three: Place the roasted pine nuts, basil leaves, olive oil, water and lemon juice in a blender and blend thoroughly.

Step four: Pour the contents of the blender into the frying pan. Add the chopped tomatoes and salt at this point. Cook on low heat until the pesto is warm (3-5 minutes).

Step five: Boil the pasta of your choice. After straining the pasta, pour the pesto over it while the pasta is still hot. Serve while warm. If needed, the pesto can be reheated at low heat.

Vegetarian Chili
(serves 4-5)

1 chopped onion
4 cloves crushed garlic
2 T ghee (clarified butter)
3 T chili powder
28 oz. tomato sauce
2 cups cooked pinto beans
2 cups cooked lentils
2 cups cooked kidney beans
1 cup grated carrots
1 cup chopped celery
1 handful finely chopped cilantro
2 chopped green onions
6 oz. frozen or fresh corn
Salt to taste

Step one: Sauté the onions in the ghee in a large soup pot on medium heat until they are translucent. Add in the garlic and chili powder. Stir for a minute, then add the tomato sauce.

Step two: Cook on high heat stirring often for about 3 minutes.

Step three: Add the beans, carrots and celery and lower the heat to a simmer. Cook until the carrots and celery are done and the beans are hot.

Step four: Salt to taste, and add the cilantro and green onions just before serving.

Tofu, Vegetable and Cashew Stir-fry
(serves 4-5)

2 T ghee (clarified butter)
1 chopped onion
6 cloves of crushed garlic
2 inches peeled, shredded ginger
1 lb. block of firm tofu, cubed
1/2 cup tamari
3 T maple syrup
1 cup whole cashews
1 head of chopped broccoli flowers
1 chopped red bell pepper

Step one: Sauté the onion in the ghee on medium heat until translucent. Add in the tofu and continue to sauté until the tofu is slightly golden brown.

Step two: Add in the tamari, maple syrup, garlic, cashews and bell pepper. Cook for five minutes, then add the broccoli and cook until the broccoli is soft.

Step three: Squeeze the juice from the shredded ginger into the stir-fry, then turn the heat off.

Chana Dal
(serves 4-5)

2 cups of chana dal (may need to purchase at an Indian grocery store)
7 cups water
2 T ghee (clarified butter)
½ cup water
6 cloves of crushed garlic
2½ inches of shredded ginger root
2 chopped carrots
1½ T coriander
1 T garum masala (may need to purchase at an Indian grocery store)
2 t turmeric
1½ t salt

Step one: Check the chana dal for stones, then wash it well. Cook on high until boiling, then reduce to a medium/high heat and continue to cook until the bean is soft, but retains its shape. This will take about one hour. If there is still water remaining when you are done cooking the dal, drain it off. While the dal is cooking you can prepare the rest of the dish.

Step two: Place the ghee, spices, carrots and crushed garlic in a frying pan and sauté for a minute or two, then add ½ cup of water and continue to cook until the carrots are soft. Add the contents of the frying pan to the dal when the dal is done cooking. Squeeze the juice from the shredded ginger into the dal.

Mattar Paneer
(serves 5-6)

8 to 10 large tomatoes
1 lb. bag of frozen peas
Paneer from 1 gallon of whole milk (*directions are provided on page 368)
2 inches of shredded ginger
6 cloves crushed garlic
2 T ghee (twice)
1 chopped onion
2 T of coriander powder
1½ T garum masala
1 T turmeric
¼ t black pepper
2 t salt

Step one: Cut the paneer into cubes and place them on baking sheet oiled well with ghee (about 2 T). Bake at 350 degrees until slightly golden brown (about 15 minutes). Stir the paneer with a spatula about half way through so as to cook the cubes more evenly.

Step two: Boil the whole tomatoes for about 10 minutes or until peel starts to split. Run the tomatoes under cold water to cool them, and then remove the peels from the tomatoes. Blend them until they are smooth in a blender.

Step three: Sauté the onions in the ghee until translucent. Add in the spices and garlic, followed by the tomatoes and peas.

Step four: Cook on medium heat until peas are soft. Add the paneer squares, and squeeze the juice from the shredded ginger into the dish.

Note: Serve over rice.

Tofu Burgers
(serves four people, makes 6 patties)

1 lb. block of firm tofu
½ cup oatmeal (uncooked)
3 T almond butter or tahini
2 to 3 T tamari (according to taste)

Step one: Place all ingredients in a food processor; mix lightly by using the pulse button approximately 20 times. Do not make into a pudding. To mix by hand, crumble tofu into crumbs, then mush other ingredients into burgers with a potato masher or knead with hands until an even consistency.

Step two: Form tofu mix into patties by hand. (3/4 of an inch thickness and 4 inches in diameter is a good suggested size.)

Step three: Sauté in a small amount of olive oil five minutes on each side over a medium heat.

Dinners

Lentil Soup
(serves 4-5)

1½ cups lentils
7 cups water
2 peeled and cubed yukon gold potatoes
2 T ghee (clarified butter)
6 cloves crushed garlic
1 bunch of red chard
1 chopped onion
3 T Italian seasoning
2 T chili powder
1 T coriander
1 pinch cayenne
3 to 4 chopped tomatoes
1 handful finely chopped parsley
4 stalks chopped green onion
1½ t salt

Step one: Wash the lentils then cook on medium/high heat in about 7 cups of water until done. This should take 45 minutes to an hour. Add the cubed potatoes to the lentils after they have been cooking for about 25 minutes.

Step two: While the lentils are cooking, sauté the onions in the ghee until translucent. Add the chard, garlic and all of the spices along with ½ cup of water. Cover and cook until the chard is soft, stirring occasionally. Add all of this to the lentils once the lentils and potatoes are done cooking.

Step three: Add the tomatoes, green onions and parsley. Keep the soup warm until serving.

Note: Serve with fresh sliced avocado.

Mung Bean Soup
(serves 5-6)

2 cups split mung beans
8 cups water
1 cup water
2 T ghee (clarified butter)
6 cloves crushed garlic
2 inches shredded ginger
1 chopped onion
1 bunch chopped red chard
3-4 chopped tomatoes
1 T turmeric
1½ T coriander
1 t cumin
¼ t black pepper
2 t salt

Step one: Check mung beans for stones, then wash and place in 8 cups of water. Cook on medium/high heat for 45 minutes to an hour, or until done.

Step two: Sauté onions in ghee on medium heat until translucent. Add all of the spices. Then add the chard and garlic along with 1 cup of water. Cover the frying pan and allow chard to steam until it is soft. Add all of this to the mung beans when they are done cooking.

Step three: Add the tomatoes and squeeze the juice from the shredded ginger into the soup. Add water to the beans, if necessary, to make the soup the desired consistency. The soup will thicken as it cools.

Toor Dal
(serves 4-5)

1½ cups toor dal (may need to purchase at an Indian grocery store)
5½ cups water
1 red onion chopped
7 cloves crushed garlic
2 inches shredded ginger
4 tomatoes chopped
1 bunch cilantro chopped
2 T ghee (clarified butter)
2 T coriander
1 T turmeric
1 T cumin
½ t Hing (Asafoetida powder) optional (may need to purchase at an Indian grocery store)
½ t ground black pepper
pinch of cayenne
1½ t salt

Step one: Check the toor dal for stones, then wash and place in 5 ½ cups of water. Cook on high until the water is boiling, then lower to a medium/high heat and continue to cook until the bean is soft. The total cooking time should be about 45 minutes to an hour.

Step two: Sauté the onions in the ghee until they are translucent. Add in all of the spices and the garlic along with ½ cup of water. Sauté for another 5 minutes, adding the tomatoes in about half way through this time.

Step three: Add the contents of the frying pan to the toor dal. Squeeze the juice of the ginger into the dal and add the chopped cilantro.

Toor Dal with Mango
(serves 4-5)

1½ cups toor dal (may need to purchase at an Indian grocery store)
6 cups water
2 inches shredded ginger
6 cloves crushed garlic
2 T ghee (clarified butter)
1 handful cilantro finely chopped
2 mangoes peeled and cubed
2 T sugar
1 T whole cumin seeds
10 whole cloves
2 t salt

Step one: Check the toor dal for stones, then wash and place in 6 cups of water. Cook on high until the water is boiling, then lower to medium/high heat and continue to cook until the bean is soft. The total cooking time should be about 45 minutes to an hour.

Step two: Heat up the ghee in a small frying pan on medium heat, when the ghee is hot, add the cloves. After the cloves have cooked for two to three minutes, remove the cloves from the ghee with a spoon. After removing the cloves, return the ghee to the heat. When the ghee is hot, add the whole cumin seeds and allow them to roast until they are golden brown (should take about 60 seconds; do not burn). Add the garlic and pour the whole mixture into the toor dal.

Step three: Add the sugar, salt, mango, cilantro and the juice from the shredded ginger to the dish.

Notes: This can be served over rice or by itself. If no mango is available just add a little more sugar to taste.

Coconut Vegetables
(serves 4-5)

2 14 oz. cans of coconut milk
2 T ghee (clarified butter)
1 chopped onion
2 heads of chopped broccoli flowers
3 cubed yukon gold potatoes
2 chopped carrots
1 chopped red bell pepper
1 large handful snow peas (cut in half)
½ lb firm tofu
6 cloves crushed garlic
2 inches shredded ginger
1 T turmeric
1 T coriander
1/8 t of red curry paste or a pinch of cayenne
¼ t ground black pepper
1 t salt

Step one: Sauté the onion in the ghee on medium heat until translucent. Add the potatoes and ½ cup of water. Cover with a lid and cook this until potatoes begin to soften (about 10-15 minutes). Stir occasionally to keep from sticking.

Step two: Add all of the spices with another ½ cup of water and stir them in. Add the carrots, tofu, bell pepper and garlic. Allow to cook for about five minutes, then add the broccoli flowers, snow peas and coconut milk. Cover and cook until all of the vegetables are soft, but not soggy (this should take about 10 more minutes).

Step three: Add the juice from the shredded ginger.

Note: Serve by itself, or over rice or noodles for a heavier meal.

Cream of Vegetable Soup
(serves 4-5)

2 T ghee (clarified butter)
6 cups water
3 yukon gold potatoes, peeled and cubed
1 onion quartered
2 carrots
2 heads chopped broccoli flowers
1 bunch kale coarsely chopped
1 bunch red chard coarsely chopped
8 whole cloves of garlic
2 inches of finely diced ginger
1½ T whole cumin seeds
½ t black pepper
2 t salt

Step one: Place all vegetables, including the garlic and ginger, in a pot with the 6 cups of water. Cover with a lid and cook on high heat until all of the vegetables are soft (about 25 min).

Step two: Heat up the ghee in a small frying pan. When the ghee is hot, add the whole cumin seeds and allow them to roast to a golden brown color (about 60 seconds; do not burn). Immediately add the contents of the frying pan to the vegetables.

Step three: Ladle all of the vegetables into a blender and blend them until they are smooth and creamy. You will have to refill the blender a few times depending on the size of the blender.

Step four: Pour the soup back into a pot and add the salt and pepper.

Vegetable Stir-fry
(serves 3-4)

1 T ghee (clarified butter)
1 chopped onion
6 cloves of crushed garlic
2 inches peeled, shredded ginger
1 head of chopped broccoli flowers
1 chopped red bell pepper
1 bunch chopped red chard
1 chopped portabella mushroom
1 large handful snow peas
2 T coriander
1 T cumin
salt to taste

Step one: Sauté the onion in the ghee on medium heat until translucent.

Step two: Add garlic and all of the spices along with ½ cup of water. Continue to sauté for 1-2 minutes then add in all of the vegetables except for the snow peas and the broccoli flowers.

Step three: After the other vegetables have cooked for about 10 minutes, add in the broccoli flowers and the snow peas. Cook until all vegetables are soft (should be another 10 minutes). Salt to taste.

Note: This will be excellent served over rice with White Tiger sauce (recipe on page 369).

Desserts

Blackberry Cobbler

Topping
¾ cup unbleached flour or whole wheat pastry flour
¼ cup quick oats
¼ cup butter
¼ cup chopped almonds
¼ t salt
½ t cinnamon
½ t vanilla
2 T maple syrup
½ cup sugar
2 T water

Crust
1 cup unbleached flour or whole wheat pastry flour
4 T butter (half a stick)
2 T water

Filling
4 cups blackberries
1 cup sugar
4 T flour
1 T lemon juice
small amount of grated organic lemon or orange peel
1 t cinnamon
½ t vanilla

Step one: Preheat oven to 350 degrees and butter a pie dish.

Step two: Prepare the crust. Add small amounts of water (2 to 3 T should be enough) to the flour and butter while mashing together with hands, until the mixture is an even consistency, and sticks to itself without being overly wet. Roll out the crust with a rolling pin so that it is large enough to cover the pie pan, then place it in the pie pan. Press the crust down where necessary to form it to the shape of the pie pan.

Step three: Prepare the topping. Place all of the ingredients in a mixing bowl and mash together with hands. Add a small amount of water (2 to 3 T) until the topping sticks a little to itself in clumps. It should be a crumbly consistency with clumps of various sizes.

Step four: Prepare filling. Gently mix all of the ingredients together in a mixing bowl. Transfer the contents onto the crust in the pie pan.

Step five: Crumble the topping evenly over the fruit so that it is covered. Place in the oven and bake for 30-40 minutes. Remove the pie when you see bubbles from the fruit and the topping is golden brown.

Cherry Cobbler

Topping
¾ cup unbleached flour or whole wheat pastry flour
¼ cup quick oats
¼ cup butter
¼ cup chopped almonds
¼ t salt
½ t cinnamon
½ t almond extract
½ t vanilla
2 T maple syrup
½ cup sugar
2 T water

Crust
1 cup unbleached flour or whole wheat pastry flour
4 T butter (half a stick)
2 T water

Filling
4 cups cherries
1 cup sugar
4 T flour
1 T lemon juice
small amount of grated organic lemon or orange peel
1 t cinnamon
½ t almond extract
½ t vanilla

Step one: Preheat oven to 350 degrees and butter a pie dish.

Step two: Prepare the crust. Add small amounts of water (2 to 3 T should be enough) to the flour and butter while mashing together with hands, until the mixture is an even consistency, and sticks to itself without being overly wet. Roll out the crust with a rolling pin so that it is large enough to cover the pie pan, then place it in the pie pan. Press the crust down where necessary to form it to the shape of the pie pan.

Step three: Prepare the topping. Place all of the ingredients in a mixing bowl and mash together with hands. Add a small amount of water (2 to 3 T) until the topping sticks a little to itself in clumps. It should be a crumbly consistency with clumps of various sizes.

Step four: Prepare filling. Gently mix all of the ingredients together in a mixing bowl. Transfer the contents onto the crust in the pie pan.

Step five: Crumble the topping evenly over the fruit so that it is covered. Place in the oven and bake for 30-40 minutes. Remove the pie when you see bubbles from the fruit and the topping is golden brown.

Fruit Bread

Dough
1 cup water
2 t yeast
3 T maple syrup
½ t salt
2½ cups flour (mix whole wheat & unbleached)

Mixed fruit
1 cup date paste
1 cup apples, chopped
1 cup raisins, chopped
½ cup dried papaya, chopped
½ cup dried pineapple, chopped
2 t ground cardamom
2 t orange zest
2 t lemon zest
1 t vanilla
1 T lemon juice
1 T orange juice

Step one: Dissolve the yeast in water and let it rest a few minutes.

Step two: Stir in the syrup and salt into the water and yeast.

Step three: Add the flour to the liquid and knead for 10 minutes. Cover, and let rise in a cool place for 2 hours.

Step four: Fold mixed fruit into dough. Lightly butter a bundt pan and line with minced pecans or sesame seeds. Cover and let rise in a cool place for 3 hours. Bake at 350 for 1 hour.

Extras

Chai (spiced milk)
(makes 2 cups)

1 cup of milk
1 cup of water
½ inch fresh ginger root
1 pinch saffron
4 whole pods of cardamom
2 T sugar
1 T black tea

Step one: Place two pots on the stove. Pour water into one pot. Pour milk into another pot. Cook both pots on high heat. Watch to make sure that the milk doesn't boil over.

Step 2: Peel and grate ½ an inch of ginger into the pot of water.

Step 3: Crush a pinch of saffron with a mortar and pestle. Add the saffron to the milk. Use a small amount of water or the 2 T of sugar that you will need to help get the saffron that will stick to the bottom of the mortar. Add the sugar or water to the milk.

If you didn't already add the 2 T of sugar, do so now.

Step 4: The water should be boiling by now. If so, add the black tea. Be sure that the water is boiling before adding the tea.

Step 5: Pour the contents of the pot that has the water into the pot that has milk.

Step 6: Crush about 4 whole pods of cardamom with a mortar and pestle. Add to the milk.

Step 7: Allow the chai to come to a boil, then quickly remove from the heat, and strain through a fine strainer so as to filter out the tea and herbs.

Ghee (clarified butter)

Step one: Place butter in a pot (4 lbs. of butter will make a good supply of ghee) and heat on medium heat.

Step two: Milk solids will start to rise to the top and should be skimmed off. Some will solidify on the bottom of the pot. This is OK, too. Do not allow the solids on the bottom to burn. If they start to turn golden brown, turn the heat off.

Step three: When all of the milk solids have been either skimmed off or settled to the bottom, pour the ghee into another pot. Be careful to leave out the milk solids from the bottom of the original pot. Use a fine strainer if you wish to be extra careful.

Step four: When the ghee has cooled, pour it into storage containers. I recommend glass jars.

Notes: Ghee does not require refrigeration and will not go bad. If it does produce mold, then it was not cooked long enough. It may solidify, or it may stay liquid, depending on its environment.

Carrot Juice

1 pound of carrots
1 apple
3 leafs of romaine lettuce

Note: Fresh juice enzymes are oxidized (used up) within 8-12 minutes after the time the juice is made. If you must store your juice, keep it in an air-tight container stored in a cool, dark place.

You will need to follow the directions given by the manufacturer of your juicer for the proper preparation of the ingredients prior to juicing.

Paneer (fresh cheese)

1 gallon whole milk
1 or 2 lemons

Step one: Bring to a boil a gallon of whole milk.

Step two: Turn the heat off, then add the juice of two to three lemons. Use only enough that you see the milk separate out into curds and whey. If it is not separating, you haven't added enough, but if you add too much, the curds will start to taste like lemon.

Step three: Bring the curds and whey to a boil again. Strain the curds out from the whey using a cheese cloth.

Step four: Lay the paneer out in-between two cutting boards, with a towel on each cutting board lined with cheese cloth, so that the paneer doesn't stick to the towels. Place something heavy on top of the top cutting board and put in the refrigerator to cool. Leave it like this for at least 15 minutes; this will press the paneer flat. After the paneer is flattened, it can be cut into cubes.

Note: Paneer can be stored in a clean, airtight container and refrigerated for up to 3-5 days before using. It is best to use the paneer within 24 hours.

White Tiger Sauce
(makes 2 cups)

½ cup sesame seeds
½ cup water
3 T rice vinegar
½ t toasted sesame oil
2 T of honey
3 crushed garlic cloves
2½ inches of peeled and shredded ginger
3 T tamari

Step one: Toast sesame seeds in oven at 350 degrees for about 15 minutes, or until lightly browned.

Step two: Use a blender to turn the toasted sesame seeds into a powder.

Step three: Add other ingredients to the blender and blend until smooth.

Note: This sauce is excellent on sautéed vegetables and on grains.

Vegetarian Gravy
(makes 3 cups)

1 T butter or ghee (clarified butter)
1 chopped onion
3 garlic cloves chopped
2 cups vegetable broth
2 T arrowroot powder
2 cups sautéed mushrooms (optional)

Step one: Sauté the onion and garlic on medium heat until they begin to brown.

Step two: Place onions and garlic in a blender. Add in the arrowroot and vegetable broth.

Step three: Return contents of the blender to the frying pan. Add the sautéed mushrooms at this point if you want them. Cook on medium heat until the gravy thickens, stirring occasionally.

Honey Dijon Dressing
(makes about 1/3 cup)

1 T cider vinegar
1 T balsamic vinegar
1 ½ t Dijon mustard
1 clove garlic, minced
1 T honey
4 T olive oil
½ t salt
Dash pepper

Combine first five ingredients in a blender and process until smooth. While the machine is running, drizzle in olive oil (which will cause the dressing to get thicker). Season with salt and pepper.

Three Bean Salad
(serves 4-5)

2 cups kidney beans, cooked tender but not soggy
2 cups garbanzo beans, cooked tender, not soggy
2 cups green beans, 1 inch segments, cooked tender
1 cup red onions, sliced in finely
1/2 cup parsley leaves, chopped

Dressing
½ cup olive oil
¾ cup balsamic vinegar
2-3 cloves garlic, crushed
½ t salt
1 T honey

Step one: Mix beans, onion and parsley together.

Step two: Mix together all ingredients for the dressing in a blender. Pour dressing over the beans onion and parsley and toss.

Index

A

Aconite 158, 159, 160
Advanced Relaxation 186, 191, 204
Alternate nostril breathing 174, 175, 176, 177
Arsenicum album 158, 160
Asanas 110, 111, 118
Avogadro, Amadoe 139
Ayurveda 17, 18, 19, 21, 22, 24, 27, 74, 79, 81, 83, 88, 89, 96, 161, 224, 231,
   233, 236, 307, 337, 338, 339

B

Bio-foodback 77
Breath 78, 79, 110, 111, 112, 173, 174, 176, 177, 215, 276, 279
Buddha 293
Buddhi 12, 14, 254
Butyric acid 337, 338

C

Calcarea carbonicum 158, 160, 161, 162
Chai 84, 90, 309, 367
Chernin, Dr. Dennis 142, 143, 147
Chitta 243
Compassion 32
Conscience 12, 33, 254, 256, 267, 268, 269, 273, 287, 302
Contemplation 241, 248, 249, 250, 251, 252, 253, 254, 256, 258, 259
Corpse pose 131, 132, 179, 180, 183, 186, 190

Endnotes

1   Tao Te Ching, Verse 33

2   Gospel of Thomas, Verse 3

3   Pandit Rajmani Tigunait Ph.D., From Death To Birth, (Honesdale, PA: Himalayan Institute Press, 1997), 29-33.

4   CDC, National Center for Health Statistics, "Prevalence of Overweight Among Children and Adolescents: United States, 2003-2004," http://www.cdc.gov/nchs/products/pubs/pubd/hestats/obese03_04/overwght_child_03.htm, accessed July 26th, 2006

5   CDC, National Center for Health Statistics, "Prevalence of Overweight Among Children and Adolescents: United States, 2003-2004," http://www.cdc.gov/nchs/products/pubs/pubd/hestats/obese03_04/overwght_adult_03.htm, accessed July 26th, 2006

6   USDA, "Vegetarian Diets," http://www.mypyramid.gov/tips_resources/vegetarian_diets.html, accessed July 26th, 2006

7   John Robbins, The Food Revolution, (York Beach, ME: Conari Press, 2001), 292.

8   Rhett A Butler, "Deforestation in the Amazon," Mongabay. com, http://rainforests.mongabay.com/amazon/amazon_destruction. html#cattle accessed July 26th, 2006

9   John Robbins, The Food Revolution, (York Beach, ME: Conari Press, 2001),266.

10   C Zoumas-Morse et al, "Children's patterns of acronutrient intake and associations with restaurant and home eating," J Am Diet Assoc Vol. 101 (2001): 923-925.

11   A Aljada, et al, "Increase in intranuclear nuclear factor kappaB and decrease in inhibitor kappaB in mononuclear cells after a mixed meal: evidence for a proinflammatory effect," Am J Clin Nutr Vol. 79, No.4 (April 2004):682-90.

12   "Summary of Edible Nuts for Aflatoxins," http://www.food. gov.uk/multimedia/pdfs/summarynuts.pdf, accessed July 26th, 2006

13   Mayoclinic.com, "Caffeine content of common beverages," http://www.mayoclinic.com/print/caffeine/AN01211, accessed July 26th, 2006

14   Anne Underwood and Jerry Adler, "Diet and Genes," Newsweek (January 17, 2005): 40-48.

15   Rudolph Ballentine, M.D., Transition to Vegetarianism, (Honesdale PA: Himalayan Institute Press, 1987), 223.

16   Rudolph Ballentine, M.D., Transition to Vegetarianism, (Honesdale PA: Himalayan Institute Press, 1987), 224.

17   FM Nagengast, IP Van Munster, "The role of carbohydrate fermentation in colon cancer prevention," Scan J Gastroenterol Suppl Vol. 200 (1993):80-6.

18   J Jacobs, et al, "Treatment of acute childhood diarrhea with homeopathic medicine: a randomized clinical trial in Nicaragua," Pediatrics Vol. 93, No. 5 (May, 1994): 719-725.

19   D Reilly, et al, "Is Homeopathy a Placebo Response? Controlled Trial of Homeopathic Potency, with Pollen in Hayfever as Model," Lancet (October, 1986): 881-86.

20   H Frei and A. Thurneysen, "Treatment for hyperactive children: homeopathy and methylphenidate compared in a family setting," British Homeopathic Journal, Vol. 90, No. 4 (1991):183-8.

21   Blair Lewis, Happiness the Real Medicine and How it Works, (Honesdale, PA: Himalayan Institute Press, 2005), 77-81,108.

22   Blair Lewis, Happiness the Real Medicine and How it Works, (Honesdale, PA: Himalayan Institute Press, 2005), 110-115.

23   "Famous Nappers," http://thewisdomofdreams.com/Famous_Nappers.html, accessed July 26th, 2006

24   Swami Rama, Path of Fire and Light Volume 2, (Honesdale, PA: Himalayan Institute Press, 1988), 180-181.

25   John 11: 9-10 (King James Version of the Bible)

26   MC Cohen, et al, "Meta-analysis of the morning excess of acute myocardial infarction and sudden cardiac death," Am J Cardiol Vol. 79, No. 11 (1997):1512-6.

27   GE Rivard, et al, "Circadian time-dependent response of childhood lymphoblastic leukemia to chemotherapy: a long-term follow-up study of survival," Chronobiol Int Vol.10, No.3 (1993):201-4.

28   MW Millar-Craig, et al, "Circadian variation of blood pressure," Lancet Vol. 1 (1978):795-7.

29   MH Smolensky, "Medical chronobiology: concepts and applications," Am Rev Respir Dis Vol. 147, No. 6, Pt. 2 (1993):S2-19

30   Pandit Rajmani Tigunait Ph.D., Seven Systems of Indian Philosophy, (Honesdale, PA: Himalayan Institute Press, 1983), 247.

31   Philippians 4:8 (King James Version of the Bible)

32   Dhammapada, Chapter 1: Verse 5

33   Matthew 5:44 (King James Version of the Bible)

ir's
ll: 214-725-1644

Center for Health and Healing
Located in the Pocono Mountains near Honesdale, PA

Ayurvedic Rejuvenation
Revitalize body, mind and soul. Based on our physician's initial consultation, you'll receive a constitution-specific program of therapeutic massage, yoga therapy, dietary counseling, biofeedback, and relaxation training.

Pancha Karma
Relax in our chalet-style guesthouse surrounded by beautiful wooded grounds. Enjoy traditional Ayurvedic therapies that gently cleanse and purify your body and mind.
- Physician Consultation
- Cleansing Diet
- Daily Steam Therapy & Ayurvedic Massage
- Other Cleansing Techniques as Prescribed
- Hatha Yoga & Meditation Instruction
- Lifestyle Recommendations

Contact Information
Center for Health and Healing
952 Bethany Turnpike
Honesdale, PA 18431
570-253-5551, ext. 3100
Email: chh@Himalayan Institute.org
Web: www.HimalayanInstitute.org